HANDBOOK OF DEMENTIA CARE

Handbook of Dementia Care

JEAN M. STEHMAN, M.A., A.C.C.

GERALDINE I. STRACHAN, R.N., M.S.N.ED.

JOY A. GLENNER

GEORGE G. GLENNER, M.D.

JUDITH K. NEUBAUER

THE JOHNS HOPKINS UNIVERSITY PRESS BALTIMORE AND LONDON

For ordering information, please write to:

The Johns Hopkins University Press, Marketing Department,

2715 N. Charles Street, Baltimore, MD 21218.

Institutions may qualify for discounts.

This book was prepared under the propriety of the

George G. Glenner Alzheimer's Family Centers, Inc.

The Johns Hopkins University Press

2715 North Charles Street

Baltimore, Maryland 21218-4319

The Johns Hopkins Press Ltd., London

LIBRARY OF CONGRESS CATALOGING-IN-PUBLICATION DATA

Handbook of dementia care / Jean M. Stehman . . . [et al.].

      p.   cm.

   Includes bibliographical references.

   ISBN 0-8018-5277-3 (pbk. : alk. paper)

   1. Dementia—Patients—Care. 2. Dementia—Nursing. I. Stehman,

Jean M.

   RC521.H35   1996

   616.8'3—dc20   95-44909

A catalog record for this book is available from the British Library.

To George G. Glenner, M.D. (1927–1995)

beloved founder of the four Alzheimer's Family Centers and the School of Dementia Care, who has left us with a determination to carry on his legacy of providing specialized loving care of Alzheimer patients and supportive services for their families. Because he believed it was urgent to share the wealth of information we have all learned from our daily experience in making the difference for this special population, the School of Dementia Care was born. We share "Dr. G"'s zest for humane care with love in our hearts for his indomitable spirit.

Contents

Preface

In 1982, the George G. Glenner Alzheimer's Family Centers, Inc., established one of the first adult day care centers in the United States for patients with Alzheimer disease and other types of dementia. The organization now has four adult day centers and the School of Dementia Care. High-quality therapeutic care based on accurate, ongoing assessment of each individual patient has always been the centers' philosophy. The term *patient* rather than *client* or a similar label is used at the centers and throughout this handbook to refer to a person with dementia. We use this term because Alzheimer disease is a medical diagnosis, and psychotropic medications are often used to control symptoms. A registered nurse is on duty all day at each of the centers. The nurse is in contact with patients' attending physicians and, through the centers' affiliation with the University of California San Diego School of Medicine, can consult with physicians at the university.

The School of Dementia Care was founded in 1987. It is a licensed California postsecondary school and provides continuing medical education for physicians through its affiliation with the University of California Office of Continuing Medical Education. It is approved to provide CEUs by the Board of Registered Nurses and the California Department of Health Services Division of Certification for Nurse Assistants. Its courses are approved by the California Department of Social Services Division of Community Care Licensing for Residential Care Facilities for the Elderly and the Board of Nursing Home Examiners. It has approved training programs for certified nurse assistants and certified home health aides.

This material was originally written in 1989 at the request of the California Department of Social Services Division of Community Care Licensing, San Diego County, for use in a Training Series on Dementia for the administrators and staff of residential care facilities for elderly persons. New State of California legislation now requires extensive initial and ongoing training for the administrators of these facilities. Before designing the training manual and the series format, the staff of the School of Dementia Care visited many facilities and discussed training needs with their staffs.

Since 1989, over one thousand people have attended the Training Series on Dementia. Even at the very first session, professionals from nursing facilities as well as residential facilities were in attendance. The material has been revised several times to meet the needs of an ever-increasing range of professional care providers. It has been widely praised by class members in the full range of long-term care professions. It has also been used in many other types of dementia education programs and as the basic manual in the dementia care portion of the School of Dementia Care's Dementia Care Specialist/Certified Nurse Assistant/Certified Home Health Aide Program.

Introduction

Alzheimer disease affects as many as one out of every six people over the age of sixty-five and at least one out of every four people over the age of eighty. It is the most common of the dementing illnesses: more than 60 percent of those with dementia have Alzheimer disease. Alzheimer disease is not normal aging, and there is still no proven treatment or cure available.

Persons with dementia are deprived of the most basic pleasures that give life meaning: active involvement in purposeful activity, shared experiences, and memories. As their disease progresses, dementia patients become unable to perform and enjoy simple tasks. Appreciating flowers, picking them, and putting them in a vase of water, or thinking about the day ahead and choosing and putting on appropriate clothing in the morning, become tasks far beyond them. Assisting these persons in rejoining life can seem like a hopeless task. However, it does not have to be so.

A well-trained care provider with knowledge of the symptoms of a dementing illness and how to deal with them can make an amazing difference. With patience, genuine caring, and interest in dementia patients as individuals, care providers can help most patients enjoy and participate in life again. The rewards for a successful caregiver are the patient's smile and the sometimes fleeting look of awareness, appreciation, and enjoyment. This response may seem insignificant, but when it comes from a previously unresponsive, passive patient, caregivers can feel that they have done wonders—and they have!

Trained, caring professional care providers can make a difference in dementia patients' lives through therapeutic programing. Therapeutic programing is defined as:

1. careful initial and ongoing assessment of each patient's weaknesses, remaining strengths, and needs; and
2. the design and implementation of individualized programs of care based in the assessment process, with the goal of maximizing each patient's remaining strengths.

The Omnibus Budget Reconciliation Act of 1987 (OBRA) mandates this quality of care for all residents of nursing facilities nationwide. The provision of such high-quality individualized programing should be the goal of all long-term care agencies, not just nursing facilities, and it is essential for all patients with Alzheimer disease or another dementia.

It is essential because dementia patients have difficulty evaluating their own needs and choosing appropriate activities, even in the earliest stages. If left to their own devices, they may sit, pace aimlessly, wander away, rummage, or develop other, more severe and potentially harmful behaviors. Once begun, these behaviors can be difficult to control. Patients are then often transferred to a higher level of care and may be physically or chemically restrained. This lack of meaningful activity or participation in harmful activity produces an excess disability that could have been eliminated or reduced through therapeutic programing.

The *Handbook of Dementia Care* is a useful reference for anyone providing long-term care for dementia patients. It emphasizes that trained professionals can and must design and implement therapeutic programs with the goal of maximizing patients' functioning. The therapeutic program should, quite simply, help dementia patients "feel good" in every sense of the term, including:

1. feeling good about themselves and feeling comfortable and secure with others around them;
2. feeling well physically;
3. feeling comfortable, safe, and confident in the physical environment;
4. feeling motivated, confident, and content in ongoing involvement in the normal activities of daily life.

The Content of the Handbook

This handbook is a guide for establishing a therapeutic program of care for dementia patients in any type of long-term care setting, including day care, home care, residential care, assisted living, and nursing facilities. It is divided into six modules. Each module covers a specific aspect of care for dementia patients, and *each one is designed to be complete in itself.* Since the modules may be used independently, each one is paginated independently.

Each module consists of an outline and accompanying handouts. The outline format was chosen to assist readers in understanding the progression of the material. The handouts are also useful references independent of the outlines.

The Glossary defines important terms used in the text. The Bibliography lists references that we recommend for further reading in the area of dementia and dementia care.

The training video for specialists, which is included with the instructor's manual, illustrates and reinforces the material presented in the handbook. Each video segment, keyed to a module, can be used to introduce the module or to review the material covered.

Who Can Use and Benefit from the Handbook?

This material has been used by professionals from the entire range of long-term care agencies. Further, family members have stated that they found the material beneficial, since every attempt has been made to present it in lay terms. The handbook, or segments of it, have been used by the staffs of many types of facilities, including:

skilled nursing facilities;
residential care facilities for elderly persons;
acute care facilities (including the staff of the first acute care hospital wing specifically for dementia patients in the United States);
adult day care centers;
home care and respite care agencies.

It has been adapted for use by people from different professions, including:

physicians;
nurses;
administrators of skilled and residential care facilities;
certified nurse assistants;
activity directors and assistants;
home health aides;
counseling and social services professionals.

A Preview of the Modules

MODULE I What Is Dementia? The Scientific Basis and Research

Module I provides an in-depth look at the organic changes in the brain involved in Alzheimer disease. It clarifies the term *dementia* and gives some information on other types of dementia. The basic neurological symptoms and some common strengths and needs of dementia patients are introduced. (These symptoms, strengths, and needs are covered again in Module IV, since they are primary considerations in planning a program for dementia patients.) Module I clarifies the difference between Alzheimer disease and normal aging and between behaviors exhibited by dementia patients and those with a nonorganic psychiatric diagnosis. The last portion of the module provides a look at useful assessment techniques for evaluating dementia patients and a simple care plan.

MODULE II Positive Interaction Techniques; Managing Behavioral and Physical Care Problems

Module II provides a detailed look at interaction techniques that work and why. The catastrophic reaction and the management of problem behaviors are discussed in detail, as are common physical care problems and the role of medication in the management of behavioral symptoms.

MODULE III Creating Supportive Physical Environments

Module III emphasizes the role that a supportive environment can have in reducing problem behaviors and in maximizing the ability to function. Diagrams illustrate some important points.

MODULE IV Choosing and Adapting Therapeutic Activities

Module IV defines the term *activities* and focuses on how to assess an *individual's* activity needs. It emphasizes the vital role of the assessment and documentation of each individual patient's physical condition, level of severity of dementia symptoms, and retained strengths and needs in the development of a therapeutic program of care. Planning activities tailored to meet individual needs is emphasized.

This module highlights types of activities that maximize each patient's remaining strengths and needs and that avoid areas of weakness. The vital role of simplified Activities of Daily Living (ADLs) and Instrumental Activities of Daily Living (IADLs) is stressed. A guide to planning activities for individual patients is included, as well as lists of simple one-step and "no-fail" activities. (Some activity ideas for individuals listed in Module IV are listed again in Module V for groups.)

MODULE V Leading Successful Group Activities; Planning a Day of Activities

Whereas Module IV focuses on activities for the individual patient, Module V focuses on activities for groups. It discusses sources of activity ideas, the division of patients into appropriate groups, appropriate behavior interventions in the group setting, and scheduling activities for a balanced therapeutic day.

This module provides detailed activity preparation and implementation sheets, a list of sources for successful activity ideas, instructions for specific activities, possible themes for tying activities together into cohesive units (which can be helpful to early dementia patients who retain some short-term memory), and a simple daily schedule.

MODULE VI Family Dynamics; Support Systems for Caregivers

The first five modules emphasize the relationship between the care provider and the patient. Module VI emphasizes the importance of the relationship of the care provider to other professional team members, resources in the community, and the family. This module describes general types of resources available locally and lists nationally available resources.

MODULES

What Is Dementia?
The Scientific Basis
and Research

MODULE I GOAL   Class members will learn about the pathology of Alzheimer disease and about the differences between Alzheimer disease, normal aging, pseudodementia, other reversible and irreversible dementias, and nonorganic brain disorders. The importance of accurate, ongoing assessment for therapeutic programing is emphasized.

I. Alzheimer disease and other causes of dementia are not normal aging

   A. Read the definitions of Alzheimer disease and dementia in the Glossary.

   B. What *is* normal aging? (Refer to Handout I:1.)

      1. Benign forgetfulness (see Glossary) is normal aging and must not be confused with Alzheimer disease.

         a. Normal older people eventually remember the things they forget; they can adapt and compensate.

         b. Persons with Alzheimer disease cannot adapt and compensate.

      2. Active and passive aging (see Glossary)

         a. People who are actively aging compensate for age-related losses by modifying their lifestyle and habits and by staying physically and mentally active.

         b. People who are passively aging have difficulty adapting to the normal changes of aging. They may be more sedentary and display less interest in daily life.

        c. The person with Alzheimer disease loses the ability to learn and adapt and is eventually unable to compensate for age-related changes.

    C. Activities of Daily Living (ADLs) and Instrumental Activities of Daily Living (IADLs) (See Glossary and Handout I:2.)

        1. Normally functioning older people have more difficulty with ADLs and IADLs with increasing age.

        2. The chances of developing a "chronic" physical problem causing "functional limitation" or "functional disability" (see Glossary): 65 to 75 percent of persons over age eighty-five need some assistance with ADLs or IADLs (U.S. Census Bureau statistics, Nov. 1992).

        3. Alzheimer disease is chronic, will *always* become worse, and will eventually cause functional disability in all areas.

II. Defining dementia

    A. Alzheimer disease

        1. Update on current Alzheimer disease research

        2. Alzheimer disease is:

           a. a disease common to aging, but not normal aging;

           b. always incurable;

           c. always irreversible;

           d. always progressive;

           e. diagnosable only on autopsy.

        3. The damage to the brain results in neurological symptoms common to all Alzheimer patients (Handouts I:6–7).

        4. Problem behaviors are a result of these basic neurological symptoms (see Module II).

    B. "What is the difference between Alzheimer disease and dementia?"

        1. Dementia is a *syndrome.* A syndrome is the presence of a specific set of symptoms (see Handouts I:6–7).

        2. Alzheimer disease is a type of dementia (see Handouts I:3–5). The symptoms are the same or very similar in all causes of dementia, but Alzheimer disease has certain notable characteristics:

           a. It is the most common cause of dementia.

           b. It is the most common type of dementia that is *always* incurable, progressive, and lethal. Other causes are quite rare.

           c. It is familially inherited in as few as 10 percent of cases (St. George-Hyslop, 1994).

        3. Types of dementia (see Handout I:3 and specific types of dementia in the Glossary).

4. Read "The Three Stages of Irreversible and Progressive Dementia" (Handout I:8).

   a. The three stages are a general guide only.

   b. All patients with irreversible, progressive dementia have similar basic neurological symptoms, but each symptom may decline at a different rate in one individual. See the case studies (Handout I:9).

C. Differentiating the behaviors of persons with primary dementias from those of persons with other mental disorders

1. Primary dementias are characterized by the development of multiple cognitive deficits (see Handout I:6) due to physiological effects (damage to brain tissue) from:

   a. the general medical condition (e.g., Alzheimer disease);

   b. the persisting effects of a toxic substance;

   c. multiple etiologies (e.g., the combined effects of cerebrovascular disease and Alzheimer disease).

2. The hallucinations and delusions of persons with dementia may not be as extensive or elaborate as those of some patients with nonorganic mental disorders.

   a. Hallucinations and delusions of dementia patients are often gross misinterpretations of the actual environment. (Illusions are also common, but are experienced by us all. An illusion is a minor misinterpretation of the environment. For example, a large plant in a corner could momentarily be interpreted as a person.)

   b. Persons with dementia are unable to build and elaborate on the hallucinations and delusions to any great extent.

3. Dementia patients, unlike many persons with other mental disorders, usually:

   a. want and need social contact, consistently positive interactions, encouragement, and reassurance;

   b. benefit from active involvement in simplified normal daily activities, but cannot relearn and need constant, step-by-step guidance.

4. Patients with other mental disorders, unlike dementia patients, can often:

   a. remember complex recent events (have short-term memory);

   b. retain information and build on it (learn);

   c. benefit from reality-awareness therapy;

   d. know that problem behaviors are inappropriate (retain insight);

   e. modify or control some problem behaviors.

5. It is important for the professional care provider to learn the history of potential patients during an initial interview. Tools such as a preadmission or preplacement appraisal may be useful. A reliable medical

diagnosis is a must. Care providers need to realize that many potential patients may have conditions that could greatly complicate care issues. Professional care providers may wish to closely evaluate the level of care required for patients with:

    a. a history of hospitalizations for psychiatric problems;

    b. severe behavior-management problems with a previous caregiver, even if the potential patient is calm during the initial interview;

    c. a history of frequent changes of placement or caregiver;

    d. a history of needing large dosages of psychotropic medication to manage difficult behaviors.

6. The caregiver may wish to take a patient on a trial basis, especially if the safety of the patient, other patients, or the staff is in question.

7. If a patient suddenly develops more severe behavioral problems:

    a. Assess for signs and symptoms of physical illness or injury that may be undetected due to the patient's decreased cognitive state (may actually be the cause of increased behavioral problems; see Module II).

    b. Analyze the routine with all care providers involved; institute changes in behavior-management strategies as needed (see Module II).

    c. If caring for more than one person with dementia, watch for problems with other patients. The care provider may need to reconsider care if the situation is disturbing to or threatens the safety or quality of life of other patients.

    d. Collaborate with the physician to examine medication regimes and adjust as needed.

III. Accurate initial and ongoing patient assessment and documentation: The key to the therapeutic program of care

    A. To keep a patient functioning at the highest level possible, caregivers must assess each patient thoroughly, develop a plan of care based on the assessment, follow it as they continue to do assessment, and then change the plan as the patient changes. (The importance of accurate ongoing assessment is stressed throughout this manual. Assessment and documentation tools are discussed again in Module IV.)

        1. A therapeutic program (see Glossary) depends on accurate, ongoing assessment and cannot exist without it.

        2. A caregiver must determine the person's true disabilities and remaining abilities in order to eliminate "excess disability" (see Glossary) caused by the lack of appropriate care or stimulation. Refer again to the case studies (Handout I:9) for examples.

3. This is especially vital with dementia patients, because they forget how to perform tasks if they do not perform them often. They must "use it or lose it."

4. Keeping a patient functioning at the highest possible level is the best current treatment for dementia.

5. Frequent reassessment is necessary as dementia progresses.

B. Documentation and assessment forms professionals should adapt and use include the following:

1. The *preadmission appraisal,* done in an initial interview. Can good-quality care be provided? What level of care is needed?

   a. A good recent comprehensive medical report is useful for reference.

   b. How severe is the dementia? Information may be in a medical report or a behavior-rating instrument (Handout I:12), or a short mental exam can be used.

   c. Will the patient be compatible with other residents or participants in a group setting? Consider the general personality, behavior problems, and level of severity.

   d. Can appropriate physical care be provided?

2. A *physician's report and medical history* (Handout I:13). This form must be complete and always available.

3. The *social history* (Handout I:14). This should be very detailed and frequently updated. It may be possible to stimulate long-term memory if the care provider knows something about the patient's past and if the social history provides cues.

4. *Mental status and level-of-severity rating instruments,* which should be updated at least every four months. (A very basic behavior rating instrument is illustrated in Handout I:12.)

   a. Instruments are a fairly reliable double check on a care provider's own informal assessment.

   b. Caution: Scales measuring *observable* behaviors are accurate only if a caregiver is familiar with the patient. Excess disability must be identified.

5. *Daily or progress notes.* These vary in form and detail any specific incidents that need to be documented.

6. The *care plan* (Handout I:15). It summarizes the total plan of care for the patient and is based on the other documentation and assessment tools used.

   a. It must be updated as changes occur.

   b. The format consists of the problem, the goal, and the plan or approach.

Positive Interaction Techniques; Managing Behavioral and Physical Care Problems

MODULE II GOAL   Class members will understand the vital role of:

1. positive interaction techniques;
2. accurate assessment of problem behaviors and catastrophic reactions;
3. a team effort for the management or resolution of problems;
4. appropriate management of physical care problems in maintaining or establishing a therapeutic program of care.

I. Positive interaction techniques: The key to success with persons with dementia

A. Interaction techniques that succeed with dementia patients can be compared to the techniques you use to make a guest feel comfortable in your home. Here are some examples.

1. Smile.
2. Make and keep eye contact during conversation.
3. Make sure your voice is warm and friendly in tone and pitch.
4. Your facial expression and body language should show that you are friendly, relaxed, and open, not tense or reserved. (Facial muscles should be relaxed, smile should be genuine, arms and hands open. Use touch if the guest does not seem reserved.)
5. Pay attention to what your guest says; try to learn more about him or her.

6. Make sure that he or she is physically comfortable.

7. Try to assess the person's feelings, needs, and preferences and respond appropriately.

B. The techniques listed above are important to use all of the time with dementia patients because:

1. Dementia patients have great difficulty understanding and coping with their environment because of their neurological problems. It is as if they are in a new situation all of the time.

2. This difficulty causes them to feel disoriented, anxious, confused, and paranoid. They need consistent, confident, calm reassurance from others to feel calm and reassured themselves.

C. Another analogy: "You come to a party where you are to meet a friend. Other guests are talking among themselves. You look around but at first you cannot see your friend. You see no one else you know."

1. How would you feel? What would you do?

2. How would you feel and what would you do if you finally saw your friend at the far end of the room?

3. Most dementia patients have similar feelings of insecurity and anxiety most of the time because of their neurological problems.

4. They withdraw if no one familiar is around to reassure and direct them, and they are drawn to a familiar person just as anyone is in an uncomfortable or a new situation.

D. Most of the points in section I.A. have to do with body language and facial expression.

1. Over 90 percent of the meaning of a verbal message is conveyed through body language and facial expression, not words.

2. Because of their many neurological problems, this is especially true for dementia patients.

a. Persons with dementia retain the ability to understand nonverbal communication longer than they understand verbal messages.

b. To correctly identify the wants and needs of dementia patients, caregivers must constantly study and assess their patients' nonverbal communication.

E. Read "Basic Principles of Positive Interaction" (Handout II:1).

F. It is very important to keep interactions on an adult level.

1. The caregiver must think of and treat the patient as an equal and as an adult who deserves respect *all of the time, regardless of his or her behavior at the moment.*

2. Caregivers must avoid:

a. using a condescending tone of voice, words, or manner;

b. offering too much assistance, "taking over";

c. praising too much or being overly affectionate.

G. Read "Understanding and Managing the Catastrophic Reaction" and the associated cue card (Handouts II:2–3).

1. Catastrophic reactions occur because the dementia patient has great difficulty understanding and coping with the environment.

a. All of us become upset when too many things are happening at once, if there is too much to do, or if we feel someone is treating us unfairly.

b. Because dementia patients cannot understand and cope as well as cognitively normal older adults, they misinterpret things and become upset more easily. (Refer to "Common Neurological Symptoms with Dementia" and the associated "Memory Trigger" Handouts I:6–7).

c. Hallucinations and delusions can cause catastrophic reactions (see Glossary). The patient believes the hallucination or delusion is real. The caregiver should neither contradict nor agree with the patient but should reassure and distract.

2. The use of good interaction techniques helps to avoid or at least minimize catastrophic reactions.

3. Vigilant ongoing assessment helps the caregiver to spot changes in the patient's behavior that might mean a catastrophic reaction is imminent. The caregiver must try to head it off before it takes place.

H. Catastrophic reactions and behavior problems are more common at the end of the day. (See the definition of Sundowner syndrome in the Glossary.) A quiet, well lighted environment and low-key, slow-paced activity can help minimize the effects of Sundowner syndrome.

II. The management of common behavior problems of persons with dementia

A. Read "Common Behavior Problems of Persons with Dementia" (Handout II:5).

B. Read "Evaluating Behavior Problems for Effective Management" and the associated cue card (Handouts II:6–7). Relate the handouts to personal experiences with patients.

C. Read and evaluate the case studies (Handout II:8), using Handouts II:6 and II:7 as guides.

III. The physical care of persons with dementia, and the relationship between physical and behavioral problems

A. Important reminders:

1. *Always* use appropriate interaction techniques!

2. To eliminate excess disability, involve patients in self-care *as much as possible.*

3. Divide activities into basic steps. A basic step is an action requiring the retention of only one thought at a time. It does not depend on a previous step or a next step but is complete in itself.

B. Read "Medical Problems and the Person with Dementia" (Handout II:9). Dementia patients usually cannot tell the caregiver if something is physically wrong, or at least cannot describe symptoms accurately. If sudden changes in behavior occur, a physical problem should be suspected.

C. Read "Assisting the Dementia Patient with Dressing" (Handout II:10).

D. Read "Nutritional Concerns for Persons with Dementia" (Handout II:11).

1. Eating is a fairly complicated process, even though it is a habitual skill based in long-term memory. Meals must be simplified more and more as the disease progresses.

2. Overeating, undereating, and inadequate fluid intake can occur in the late second and third stages of the disease process. Monitor the intake of food and water, because patients may not recognize feeling full, hungry, or thirsty.
   a. The body's ability to process nutrients also can deteriorate as the disease progresses.
   b. Supplements can be used if the person has great difficulty eating and loses a great deal of weight.
   c. Offer water frequently.

3. Choking and difficulty swallowing become very real dangers as the disease progresses.
   a. Many patients bolt their food. They eat very rapidly and take no time to chew.
   b. In the second and third stages of the disease, the person needs constant monitoring while eating.

E. Read "Oral Care" (Handout II:12) and "The Use of Dentures and Other Assistive Devices" (Handout II:13).

F. Read "Incontinence" (Handout II:14).

1. Caregivers must remember that the person's self-respect and self-esteem are of vital importance. If the person needs assistance, the caregiver should do the following:
   a. Privately ask the person if he or she needs to use the bathroom. Always discuss problems privately.
   b. Avoid words that sound like an order. The caregiver could say, "The bathroom is free. This is a good time to go," rather than "You must go to the bathroom now."

c. Keep the toileting process as private as possible. Let the person continue to go alone as long as he or she can (evaluate for decline in skill level frequently, however). If the person needs only a little help, leave him or her once seated *if* it is safe. Then, leave the door slightly ajar and wait just outside.

d. When assisting, divide the task into simple steps and encourage the patient to do as much as possible by himself or herself.

2. Bowel and bladder problems can occur because the person may not void and urinate regularly and completely and clean properly.

a. The person may be unable to concentrate long enough to void properly.

b. The person may be unable to identify and communicate the problem and discomfort, and impactions or infections can develop.

G. Read "The Management of Sleep Disturbances Common among Persons with Dementia" (Handout II:15).

1. Nighttime wandering and rummaging are very common problems and can ruin the health of patients and family care providers, who usually have twenty-four-hour-a-day duty.

a. Darkened, quiet rooms at night may help if the problem is that the patient does not realize it is nighttime.

b. Evaluate for comfort. The person may be disoriented, be too warm or cold, or need to use the bathroom.

2. Excessive sleeping can occur because patients are unable to remain active by themselves during the day and are not involved in therapeutic activities by their care providers. Or, they may be too heavily medicated or depressed. Caregivers should problem solve with the goal of keeping patients awake for most of the day so that normal sleep patterns can develop.

3. Hallucinations and delusions are more common at night. The patient may have always been a little fearful at night and is probably having trouble interpreting the darkened environment.

a. Caregivers should assure the patient that they are taking care of the problem.

b. If the caregiver argues with patients that there is nothing wrong, patients will only be more upset and distrustful, because they are quite sure something is actually wrong.

H. Read "Assisting the Dementia Patient with Bathing" (Handout II:16). Why is bathing often so difficult?

1. Discussion: "Think about how it would feel to be bathed or showered if you had no idea what was taking place." One's modesty and pri-

vacy are invaded, and all the senses are bombarded. One's balance is precarious, and there are many complex steps in the process.

2. The caregiver must make sure that the patient maintains awareness of and confidence in what the caregiver is doing (as much as the level of functioning allows).

   a. While maintaining the patient's awareness and confidence, the caregiver should bathe or shower the person slowly, gently, and quietly, reducing excess stimulation.

   b. Caregivers should tell the patient simply what they will be doing next, speak reassuringly, and present simple steps one at a time.

   c. If bathing is really difficult, sponge bathing of one area at a time (maybe one section of the body each day), while the patient is seated on a well-waterproofed bed, may be an option.

I. The role of medications in behavior management (Handouts II:17–18)

   1. Definition of psychotropic drugs (see Glossary)

   2. Medication provides only limited help in the management of problem behaviors. The primary function of behavior-altering medication is to improve the quality of life for the patient, not to serve as a restraint. It does not substitute for consistent, appropriate interaction techniques and for involvement in an ongoing program of appropriate activity. Medication should *never* be used simply to make life easier for the professional caregiver.

   3. Watch for side effects, especially when the medication or dosage is changed.

   4. A set routine for medicating and the establishment of blood levels is vital.

      a. After evaluating the patient's behavioral patterns, the patient's physician must determine the treatment schedule.

      b. Medication administered only when a problem occurs may not be as effective.

   5. The caregiver should call the pharmacist with any questions about a medication.

Creating Supportive

Physical Environments

MODULE III GOAL Class members will gain increased understanding of the positive and negative effects the physical environment can have on the behavior and general functioning level of patients with dementia, and will learn to evaluate and make positive changes in the environment accordingly.

I. A positive, supportive environment: an essential component of maximal quality of life

   A. If we are successfully maintaining the quality of life, we "feel good." Certain positive components must be present in our lives for us to feel good. These include:

      1. positive feelings and relationships (about and with oneself, with others, and spiritually);

      2. physical well-being;

      3. satisfying work and leisure activities;

      4. a pleasant, comfortable physical environment that supports and assists in maintaining the other three components.

   B. Dementia patients need all four components for maximal quality of life, just as cognitively normal people do. The job of a therapeutic program is to assist them in maintaining these components, because they can no longer do it for themselves.

      1. All four components necessary for feeling good must be present in a

therapeutic program. If any is missing or deficient, the quality of life will suffer. For example, if patients are not provided with meaningful "work-type" and leisure activities, they become bored and restless. Friends, good health, and a pleasant environment are not enough if they have nothing to do all day.

2. The four components overlap and affect each other. For example, the physical environment is unpleasant if is cold or the furniture is uncomfortable. It affects the patients' physical well-being (they will be cold or otherwise uncomfortable), and they will not want to engage in activities or visit with friends there because of the discomfort.

3. All four components are covered throughout this manual, but each of the four is emphasized in separate modules.

   a. Positive feelings and relationships were covered in Module II.

   b. Physical health and comfort were covered in Module II.

   c. Satisfying work and leisure activities will be covered in Modules IV and V.

   d. A supportive physical environment is covered in this module—Module III.

II. Environmental changes beneficial for all older adults

   A. All of a person's senses and the ability to move about in and manage the physical environment decline with age (also see Module I). To make these age-related changes easier to deal with, older people make adaptations to their environment. For example:

      1. Older people may move into a one-level or a smaller home to make home management easier and safer.

      2. They may need to use large-print books or a magnifying lens due to poorer near vision.

      3. They may turn up the volume on the television and radio and may need to stand closer and listen more intently to speakers. They may also eventually need some type of hearing aid due to declining auditory acuity.

   B. As one sense is reduced, older people rely on the better senses more. As all senses are reduced, older adults rely heavily on multiple cues.

   C. Read "Common Sensory Problems of Aging and Environmental Modifications to Assist and Support" (Handout III:1.)

III. Why are environmental adaptations important for persons with dementia?

   A. Alzheimer disease and most related dementias are diseases of older adults. Dementia patients need the same environmental adaptations useful to any older adults. These adaptations are even more important for dementia patients, however, since they need to rely more heavily on basic senses because their cognitive abilities are declining.

1. Their decreased perception and memory of the location and function of objects, and their decreased ability to make correct judgments and reasoned choices in the environment, make functioning in everyday living extremely difficult and even dangerous.

2. If a person's only condition is Alzheimer disease or a related type of dementia, the basic senses, physical strength, dexterity, motor skills, and stamina do not usually decline any more rapidly than those of a normal older person until the last stage of the disease (see Modules I and IV). The care provider must adapt the environment so that it helps the cognitively impaired person to maximize these retained strengths.

3. The care provider must simplify the environment and maximize effective sensory cues. Persons with dementia rely even more on multiple sensory cues than do normally functioning older adults.

4. A carefully designed and controlled environment increases patients' self-confidence and self-esteem, because they can function in it more easily. It allows them more freedom. It also makes life far easier for the staff.

   a. Care providers can spend less time controlling behaviors. They do not have to constantly tell patients "No," redirect them, or take things from them.

   b. A controlled environment is an excellent behavior-management tool. It makes life easier for the care provider and patient alike.

B. There are many different ways in which the environment can help maximize patients' remaining abilities. The environmental adaptation ideas discussed in this module have been used successfully by many care providers. However, different strategies work with different patients. There are few absolute answers in any aspect of dementia care. What *can* be done is to learn what has worked for others, try the ideas, and adapt them for one's own use.

C. Ideas to be presented are generally suitable for use with patients in all types of care settings: small (board-and-care) and larger residential care settings, skilled care, day care, and private homes.

IV. Adapt ideas presented in Sections V, VI, and VII to your own care setting

A. Different types of environmental adaptation are discussed in Sections V, VI, and VII of this module. These include: maximizing general sensory stimulation in a homelike setting (V); using sensory cues to enhance patients' ability to use the environment appropriately and for orientation and wayfinding (VI); and environmental adaptations for safety and ease of surveillance (VII).

    B. Use Handout III:2 to summarize changes you may wish to make in your own care setting, based on the ideas in Sections V, VI, and VII.

V. Maximizing sensory cues in a homelike environment

    A. Maximizing sensory stimulation in a homelike setting can increase the general level of awareness, feelings of security, and general well-being. A homelike environment is widely recognized as an effective tool in therapeutic dementia care. (A homelike setting is the goal at all of our centers and is recommended by Cohen and Weisman 1991, Coons 1991, and others.)

    B. Choose furniture that is homelike and of a type familiar to patients. (Ultramodern furniture, for example, may not appeal to a majority of older patients.) Choose a variety of tables, seating types (lounge chairs, hard-backed chairs, soft low chairs, couches) and other furnishings for comfort, specific use, and homelike design.

       1. Furniture upholstery that resist stains and liquids but does not look institutional is now available.

       2. Use a variety of well-coordinated colors in furniture and bright colors for accent, not just sterile white. Aging eyes respond best to warm, bright colors.

       3. Quilts, afghans, and accent pillows of different textures and colors provide tactile and visual stimulation. (The staff must monitor rummagers, who may pick up pillows and leave them around where others can trip over them.)

       4. Be careful not to overstimulate. The use of many different bright colors and patterns can confuse or agitate.

    C. Use things that are familiar from patients' past for decoration and to provide stimulation. For example, Cohen and Weisman's book *Holding On to Home* (1991) contains a picture of a facility in a farming community. The walls are decorated with well-secured old farm and household implements familiar to the residents, most of whom have lived their entire lives in that rural community. These items provide not only visual but also tactile stimulation. They stimulate long-term memory and provide opportunities for conversation and bonding between residents. (Remember that older adults have a lower field of vision, so place wall items at an appropriate height for them and for wheelchair-bound patients.)

    D. Wallpaper increases a homelike appearance, but avoid prints that can confuse or distract. Pastels are usually best in wallcoverings over wide areas. Combine with solid painted walls in soft, related colors.

E. Display patients' artwork, but avoid clutter and overstimulation. (Use only items that look adult and that they are proud of.) If facilities are adequately staffed and use appropriate behavior interventions, displaying items will be easier. If rummaging and hoarding become a severe problem, however, try the following:

1. It may be possible to display items out of reach on a high shelf or high on a wall.

2. Try having one room as an "art room" that can be easily monitored, or use display cases.

F. Auditory stimulation is just as important as visual and tactile.

1. Music sets a mood; use it purposefully. Soft, soothing music during meals, grooming, or relaxation periods can be effective. It should *not* be used when residents must concentrate on verbal instructions or when other confusing auditory or visual stimuli are present.

2. Eliminate loudspeakers; control loud conversations between staff members or visitors, barking dogs, traffic sounds, the ringing of phones, the sounds of dishwashers and washing machines. Do not leave the television on for long periods of time; use it for selected activities only. Such extraneous auditory stimuli can be very distracting and can cause increased behavior problems and catastrophic reactions.

G. Olfactory stimulation is often overlooked. Pleasant cooking smells and fragrant plants and flowers add appropriate stimulation. Be alert to overpowering, unpleasant odors, which can disturb patients, staff, and visitors and deter potential clients.

VI. Using sensory cues to enhance patients' ability to use the environment appropriately and for orientation and wayfinding

A. Furnishings and implements for patients' use should be chosen for interest and for ease of use.

1. Patients need to be able to sit on and rise from chairs independently (Handout III:3). Chairs must glide easily. Patients' self-esteem is lowered and frustration increases if they have to ask for help every time they want to get up or sit down. A big, soft, comfortable chair that is difficult to get out of may *occasionally* be useful for patients who wander excessively. If they need rest but seem unable to stop pacing, seating them in an overly soft chair that is rather difficult to get out of can encourage them to obtain needed rest. (Be careful! The care plan must

clearly state that the chair is to be used for the patient's well-being, not for staff convenience.)

2. Tables must be the right height for use with the chairs provided.

3. Provide fairly high tables next to or in front of chairs for coffee cups, magazines, etc. High tables are more easily visible and safer than coffee tables. They must be easily visible from the chair, since the dementia patient may forget that the table is there to use.

4. Drawers should slide open easily, and shelves for patients' use should be within easy reach and not too deep, to encourage continued active participation and independence in choosing and storing their own clothing.

5. Closets should be wide and bars for clothing low enough for easy use. (Remember, install closet bars and other objects for daily use, such as mirrors and bookshelves, at a lower level for all older adults and even lower for wheelchair-bound patients.)

   a. Clothing does not have to be stored on hangers. If patients cannot use hangers anymore, place two or three bars in the closet at staggered depths and heights. Patients can then fold their clothing over the bars.

   b. To avoid confusion and rummaging, a locked closet (in the resident's room or preferably elsewhere in the building) can contain most clothing, while only a few items are kept in the resident's closet for immediate independent use.

   c. Consider ease of use when choosing implements for patients' use. Light switches on walls and on lamps, faucet handles, eating and craft utensils, and drawer, door, and cabinet knobs should be large, highly visible, and easy to use appropriately.

B. Keep carefully selected activity items out for patients' independent use. Meaningful, productive activity (e.g., simplified IADLs such as folding laundry, washing dishes, raking leaves, and sweeping) is a primary behavior-management tool and vital to optimal functioning. Patients will generally not think to engage in productive activity on their own but may occasionally do so if it is clearly visible. ("Out of sight, out of mind" is usually the situation.)

1. *Important:* Activity supplies must be organized, well labeled, and easily accessible to the staff so that appropriate activities are always readily available.

2. Select activity supplies to be left out for safety. Don't display valuable items or things that cannot be easily replaced.

3. Pets (carefully selected, cared for, and monitored!) and plants provide opportunities for independent initiation of activity.

4. Books, magazines, cards, pictures, albums, etc. (not too many), on a shelf or table can stimulate interest.

5. Carefully selected rummaging boxes (see Module IV) can be set out occasionally (vary the selection and keep only one or two out at a time).

6. Pictures or other items on walls encourage discussion and reminiscing. Any scenes from the past (Grandma Moses farm scenes would be appropriate in a rural farming area), scenes of familiar spots nearby, or pictures of animals or children are good. Avoid pictures that could be misconstrued—storms, battle scenes, sad or difficult situations. Hang pictures in locations and at a height where patients can really enjoy them. Anchor them securely.

7. Post large-print *daily* activity schedules for patients' use. At least a reminder of the day and date should be in every room used by patients. Clocks are also useful. Patients may not be able to read and remember activity schedules and remember the time, but these things act as reminders and are reassuring. (Occasionally patients become fixated on the time. Clocks should be removable in case this becomes a problem.)

8. Carefully selected music can stimulate spontaneous singing, movement to music, or even an impromptu dance.

9. Outdoors, provide raised garden beds at or just below waist height, if possible. Gardening is an activity enjoyed by many adults. Provide a variety of attractive, *safe, and nonpoisonous* plants that provide olfactory and visual stimulation. Raised garden beds are more accessible and safer for any older person, but especially for those who have problems with perception and organization of movement.

C. The design of a care setting can facilitate involvement in activity. In the residential facility floor plan in Handout III:4, the activity area and the outdoor area are visible from all patients' rooms. If activities are going on, patients will see them and are more likely to initiate involvement independently. (It helps to reduce the "out of sight, out of mind" problem.)

D. The appearance of a room or area should cue patients to its use (Handout III:5). The type, position, and contrasting color of furnishings should provide cues to what is taking place there.

1. The design of furniture should be appropriate to its use. (For instance, seating patients in soft chairs at a table for exercise is not appropriate.) The furniture should contrast in color with the floors and walls. The colors of floors, doors, and walls should contrast as well, so that patients have a clearer picture of the room boundaries.

2. The position of furniture should be appropriate to the function. For example, patients can be seated right next to someone and not be aware that the person is there, or a rousing game of ball can be going on and they can be unaware that anything is happening. Chairs should be angled toward other participants and/or toward the leader, to assist patients in retaining maximal awareness and attention span (see Handout III:5).

3. Before beginning an activity, the staff must think about the best way to position furniture and move it accordingly. The staff will need to allow extra time for moving furniture; though it needs to be stable, it should also be chosen for ease of movement by the staff.

4. Areas to be used for exercise or other large-motor activities or for cognitively demanding activities should be well lit and cheerful. Furnishings should allow for easy movement.

5. Areas for rest and relaxation or to "get away" should have softer lighting, soft and comfortable furnishings (reclining chairs, rockers), and more muted colors. In all care settings, patients should have a "quiet area" to retreat to. In residential facilities, residents who need rest may return to activities more easily and quickly if they have a quiet area to go to and relax rather than always going back to their rooms. (See Handouts III:4–5.)

6. Floor coverings and dividers can help distinguish areas in a large room divided for different uses (Handout III:5).

E. Provide patients with cues to set apart their room or their portion of a shared room in a residential care setting.

1. Shared patient rooms are often a problem. Patients find it difficult to distinguish their belongings from their roommate's or may rummage through or hoard the other person's belongings. Many residential care facilities are experimenting with private patient rooms, but of course, the cost then becomes higher and loneliness could be a problem.

2. Any patient room, single or shared, must be as homelike, safe, and accessible as possible and should contain items and furnishings from the residents' past *which still have positive associations for them.*

3. If items from home are not available, each resident should at least have furnishings that can be distinguished from those of other residents by style and/or color. Bedspreads should all be different. Bright individualized stickers on each resident's belongings can also help.

4. If rooms must be shared, familiar items can help residents distinguish their part of the room.

F. Provide cues for ease of movement and wayfinding in and between areas of a facility.

1. Avoid clutter in rooms. While patients get a cue to a room's use from

the position of the furniture (Handout III:5), a cluttered, crowded room gives no positive cues and they may refuse to enter.

   a. Meals can be a very stressful time. Crowding and noise at meals is common. Eating areas should be uncrowded and quiet. Soft background music may help if there is not too much external noise to compete with.

   b. An uncrowded space for a small group of dementia patients works best (groups of ten or fewer for meals and most activities). Simplified meals and plates and cups in a color that contrasts with the placemats and table may help orient the person and reduce confusion as well.

2. Provide space and lots of cues for easy initiation of independent large-motor activity (see Handout III:4).

   a. Patients with Alzheimer disease or other primary dementia are often still physically fit and retain strength and dexterity. Walking is the primary activity of wanderers. Specific, clearly marked wandering paths both inside and out (Handout III:4) are needed in any facility caring for dementia patients.

   b. Make sure paths are wide, have no uneven areas, and are clearly marked. Furniture should not be in the way. Avoid hanging plants that may bang heads!

   c. Avoid patterns, stripes, or squares on flooring which could look like three-dimensional barriers or holes.

   d. Avoid sharp turns and angles on the path. Lower-functioning patients who need to make a right-angle turn or to turn around and walk back on a path sometimes think they are lost because they cannot make the required turns without assistance.

   e. Any wandering path must take patients back to the same familiar spot or they may feel disoriented. In addition, out- of-doors, doors to the inside should be well marked, since patients may actually be afraid to leave the familiar inside world. Staff members may need to point out the door as they go outside, reassuring patients that they will not be left alone and will return to that door.

   f. Provide objects of interest and places to rest along indoor and out-door wandering areas.

3. Patients often have trouble finding their room or finding a bathroom. If there are many rooms in a care setting with all doors alike, and if all resident rooms are furnished and arranged in a similar way, it is no wonder that this is a problem. Ideas for easing such problems include (also see Handout III:6):

   a. Painting different hallways and doors or door frames in different colors. Bathroom doors should contrast with residents' room doors.

b. Placing arrows or lines on walls or floors, which patients can follow to get to the bathroom independently. These would be successful only with higher-functioning dementia patients, however; lower-functioning patients would be unable to grasp and retain the concept.

c. Using more than one cue to identify bathrooms. The universal symbols for men and women are often hard for dementia patients to distinguish. Try combining them with the word plus a picture of a man or woman next to the door. The word *toilet* and a picture of a toilet are also useful.

d. Using very large door numbers on or beside residents' doors.

e. Hanging individualized decorative items (such as a wreath) on or beside residents' doors.

f. Using photos along with large-print name plates (at least two inches in height) on or beside each resident's door. Photos must be clear, simple, and meaningful to each patient, however, to be effective. Patients may most readily recognize pictures of themselves when they were young.

g. Using "bio boards" next to the doors. These boards contain the name of the resident and something about him or her which has meaning. Photos are also included. These not only help residents identify their rooms but also give them topics of conversation with visitors.

h. Placing lucite display boxes next to the door. These go a step further than bio boards because they can hold three-dimensional objects that are currently meaningful to residents.

G. Consider lighting. The perceptual problems of dementia patients make good lighting especially important, since they easily misinterpret the environment.

1. Shadows or bright light glaring on floors and walls can look like holes or barriers. Shadows in corners can look like threatening figures. Dark hallways often just look too threatening to enter, since the patient cannot see in them and cannot remember what is there.

2. Use matte glass on pictures placed for patients' enjoyment. If light glares on the picture, it cannot be seen.

3. Position chairs carefully indoors and out to avoid glare. Glare can distract or even hurt the eyes, yet patients will not know to reposition their chairs appropriately. Have the primary outdoor seating area under an awning or a porch to avoid glare and to encourage more outdoor activities. It is difficult for anyone to concentrate visually on a project or to read outside in bright sunlight. In addition, patients on

some psychotropic medications may be light sensitive (they should wear hats when in direct sunlight).

VII. Adaptations of the environment for safety and ease of surveillance

    A. Dementia patients need to stay active and move about freely, yet due to their perceptual problems and lack of ability to reason well and use good judgment, the most ordinary things can be dangerous. The care provider needs to use a combination of environmental safety modifications and unobtrusive, yet *constant* surveillance to ensure safety. Without such modifications, the care provider needs to spend far more time redirecting patients. This reduces patients' self-esteem and independence.

    B. Modify the environment for safety. See the list of catalogs of adaptive supplies in Handout III:7. Hardware stores often have needed supplies. Many safety points have been mentioned in earlier sections, but below are some important additional points:

        1. Choose furnishings for safety as well as for sensory stimulation and ease of use.

           a. Avoid low tables and sharp corners. Choose seating, lamps, and tables for stability. Secure lighting cords and other electrical wiring to avoid tripping.

           b. Beds should not be too high. Consider the use of bed rails carefully. If a patient tries to climb over them, he or she may easily fall.

        2. Modify bathrooms for safety.

           a. Use nonskid flooring.

           b. Use rails on tubs and showers and beside toilets.

           c. Use raised toilet seats, if needed. (Some patients are afraid of these, however)

           d. Use hand-held showers and sturdy shower seating for ease of use and safety.

           e. Watch the water temperature! Water hot enough for dishwashing is much too hot for patients' use. Large, leverlike handles, which are easy to turn, are available (see catalogs in Handout III:7). Make sure the hot and cold symbols are easily visible.

        3. Make sure that the dimensions of exercise areas, hallways, and pathways are clearly visible and that these areas are free of obstructions.

           a. Remember to provide contrast in color between floors and walls to make boundaries more visible.

           b. Remember to provide adequate lighting without glare.

           c. Handrails should be highly visible against walls and placed wherever additional support may be needed (around corners, along ramps, always on both sides of stairs).

   d. Steps should be easily distinguishable by bright edgings or alternating colors. Eliminate steps wherever possible.

   e. Avoid anything that could trip a patient.

   • Don't use small area rugs. Anchor the edges of larger rugs securely.

   • The edges of sidewalks should be level with the grass, and sidewalks should be wide. Avoid low sidewalk edgings.

   • A small step down from one area to another can be a real danger. A small ramp offers a safer transition.

4. Control access to and interest in areas of potential danger.

   a. Use key locks or childproof latches on cabinets where patient access is a problem. Remove dangerous items from the area whenever possible.

   b. Dutch doors or half-doors with interior sliding locks can be used in areas where patients need visible access but from which they sometimes must be excluded. Such areas might include a kitchen or an outdoor area, or even an office (see Handout III:4).

   c. Fence outdoor areas (Handout III:4). Use high fences that also screen views of streets or parking areas. Physically fit dementia patients can often climb amazingly well!

   d. Block views of busy streets or parking areas by covering smaller windows not needed for light (such as panels in doors) or using blinds.

   e. Doors can be camouflaged by painting them and the doorknobs the same color as the wall, by wallpapering them, or by continuing designs on walls across door areas (see Handout III:6). (Check with licensing and fire regulations before camouflaging an exit door, however.)

   • Screens in front of doors or just covering up door handles may also be effective.

   • "Sorry, Closed," "No Entry," or even "Wet Paint" signs and portable waist-high stop sign barriers have worked in some care settings.

   f. To discourage thoughts of leaving, don't hang coats near doors. Discourage women from carrying their purses everywhere.

   g. Patient activity areas should be away from main exits (Handout III:4). Whenever possible, have visitors enter and leave out of patients' view.

   h. Don't store luggage and outdoor coats and hats in residents' rooms.

C. Adapt the environment for easy and *unobtrusive* surveillance.

1. Even the safest environment is still not absolutely secure. Patients can fall in the safest exercise area or can figure out how to leave from a well-camouflaged exit door.

2. Dementia patients cannot be left on their own, yet it is impossible and would be too invasive of privacy to hover over them all the time. Constant obvious monitoring by a care provider can agitate a patient, since no one likes to feel he or she is constantly being watched.

3. Environmental surveillance adaptations take some of the burden off care providers and free them for quality time with patients. (*Important note:* Care for dementia patients is so demanding that care providers also need time to themselves during each and every day. Even the most dedicated staff member needs a place to store belongings— and to get away from patients' reach and view for breaks *only*.)

4. Many types of specially designed security devices are available. See Handout III:8 for a short summary.

   a. Special licenses and releases are needed to keep patients in a locked facility (see Module VI).

   b. Locks that release by the use of special codes and time-delayed locks are often considered less restrictive.

   c. Alarm systems are usually permitted. Cowbells or temple bells that ring when doors are opened can provide an extremely basic type of alarm system.

   d. Care providers should check with their regulatory body before choosing any surveillance system.

5. When thinking of security, remember windows and outdoor fence gates as well as the doors of a building.

6. Alarms and locks help, but visual surveillance is also needed.

   a. Large windows can be installed between nurses' stations or offices and activity areas or hallways.

   b. When designing new facilities, position offices or nurses' stations for easy view of patient use areas. In the floor plan in Handout III:4, all patient room doors, the activity area, and the outdoor area can be seen from the office.

   c. Bathrooms used by patients must be easily monitored as well as private. The use of curtains around toilet stalls and showers instead of solid doors can enable care providers to monitor and maneuver more effectively. Don't eliminate privacy curtains, as this would be an invasion of the patient's dignity and basic privacy.

7. Outings in a van and walking are wonderful activities, but if a care provider takes patients for walks or outings away from the care setting, other staff members must always know exactly where the group is. A communication system (walkie-talkies on walks and phones in vans) is a good idea in case someone bolts or just wanders off, or in case of accident.

Choosing and Adapting

Therapeutic Activities

MODULE IV GOAL   Class members will understand the varying activity needs of individual dementia patients and will know how to meet these needs by choosing and adapting appropriate activities.

I. What are activities? Why are they important?

A See the definition of *activity* (Glossary)

B. See the definition of *therapeutic activity* (Glossary).

1. Therapeutic activity is part of a *therapeutic program* (see Glossary).
    a. A therapeutic program is accomplished by setting and working toward goals for patients based on careful assessment of their needs. Its goal is to eliminate *excess disability* (see Glossary), to help patients "feel good" in all ways.
    b. "Feeling good" involves:
        • feeling well physically and emotionally, including positive relationships with others (see Module II);
        • feeling positive about and comfortable in the physical environment (see Module III);
        • active participation in satisfying therapeutic activity (this module and Module V).
2. Therapeutic activity is *the primary treatment* in a therapeutic program for persons with dementia. This is because their primary disability is the

inability to plan, initiate, carry out, or remember activities by themselves. Caregivers must assist them throughout an activity, from beginning to end.

    a. For all human beings, involvement in worthwhile, satisfying activity *gives life meaning.*

    b. Keeping patients involved in meaningful activity is the *primary* therapy in a therapeutic program for persons with dementia. Their primary disability is the inability to plan, initiate, carry out, or remember activities by themselves. If left alone, they may just sit, become agitated or restless, or perform repetitive, meaningless activities. Patients can stay involved in life in a meaningful way if care providers assist them throughout activities, from beginning to end.

II. Choosing therapeutic activities

    A. Choose appropriate therapeutic activities for dementia patients based on careful assessment and documentation of each individual's medical history; history of interests, habits, and support systems; severity of neurological symptoms; and ability to function in daily life, including emotional state and behavior problems.

        1. Use a variety of assessment and documentation tools. *No one tool gives a complete picture of the person's actual ability to function (eliminating excess disability).*

        2. The home caregiver may need fewer formal assessment and documentation tools. Nursing facilities require extensive documentation. However, all caregivers should use some tools to obtain more accurate, objective assessments and to assist them in program planning.

        3. Patients must be evaluated on an ongoing basis. Document and plan for changes accordingly.

        4. Assessment and documentation tools useful to caregivers include the following:

           a. A social history (a sample is included in Module I). It documents past interests, any interests the patient retains, and a history of relationships and support systems.

              • Habits and preferences should also be listed. This is especially important for dementia patients, since they cannot adapt to change easily. Care facilities usually keep carefully set schedules and routines; however, it is much easier on staff members and residents alike if facilities adapt to the schedules and habits of individual residents. For example, since his retirement, Harry has always taken a daily shower after a brisk walk at 4:00 P.M. He is now moderately impaired with Alzheimer disease and has been placed in a nursing facility. If the staff expects him to bathe at 8:00 A.M. every day, they will probably have a great deal of difficulty with him during the bathing process.

- In skilled nursing facilities, this documentation is divided between the Social Services and Activities departments.

b. The *medical history* (a sample is included in Module I). It documents past and current medical conditions. Therapeutic activities can be part of a treatment program. Activities may have to be modified due to physical conditions.

c. *Daily notes* of various types. These document, usually in a narrative style, noticeable changes of any kind in the patient. A file or notebook detailing activity successes (and failures!) with individual patients is useful. Entries should be dated, since a person with progressive dementia will eventually decline in all areas.

d. *Mental status exams.* These are fairly accurate, objective assessment tools for documenting cognitive ability. They are time consuming to perform, since the caregiver must ask the patient a series of questions. However, they are useful in establishing a patient's *true* ability level. Many types are available.

e. *Various scales* to assess and document the person's performance of daily life functions, including emotional state, behavior problems, and performance of ADLs and IADLs. (One version is the behavior-rating instrument in Module I.)

- These scales rate the observed level of performance, rather than ability, and are more subjective. The caregiver must be aware that a patient's performance may fluctuate from day to day, depending on health, amount of sleep the night before, general comfort, and distractions present.

- To discover the person's true ability to function, eliminating any excess disability, the caregiver should use these scales in conjunction with the mental status assessment, medical history, social history, and daily notes.

f. The *care plan.* This details the caregiver's individualized, therapeutic plan of care for each patient. The caregiver should assess each patient on an ongoing basis and, as problems change, change the goals and approaches accordingly. (See case study, Handout IV:1.)

- Since involvement in therapeutic activity is the key to therapeutic programing, activities should be emphasized in the care plan (Handouts IV:2–3).

- Involvement in specific activities should be included as care plan goals and is an effective approach for reaching goals.

B. Different activities require different abilities, maximize different strengths, and meet different needs. Caregivers must assess what an activity can provide for patients (the goal of the activity) and match it with the goals for a patient as stated on the care plan.

C. The common neurological symptoms of progressive dementia (see Handouts I:6 and IV:4) will always get worse. The caregiver should not eliminate the stimulation of these declining abilities, however. The goal of a therapeutic program is to *keep* the patient functioning as well as possible in all areas, not to avoid the use of these skills. If the caregiver avoids them, an excess disability may be created. A dementia patient *cannot relearn* but must "use it or lose it."

1. The three stages of dementia are guides only. A person will not decline at the same rate in all skill areas.

2. Specific activities can be designed to maximize skills retained well and to minimize skills that are weak. For example, Saul retains fairly good language skills, ability to reason, short-term memory, and attention span. However, he has poor perceptual skills and is very aware of this. In a simplified version of basketball for a group of patients, Saul enjoys assisting the caregiver with scorekeeping but seldom takes a turn at the basket and does not wish to be a member of a "team."

3. When encouraging patients to use declining skills, assess and watch for decline. The patient *must not* be pushed to perform beyond his or her skill level. This is devastating to self-esteem and can cause catastrophic reactions. Dementia patients cannot relearn. *Activities must be designed for success.*

D. Though patients with progressive dementia eventually decline in all areas, they retain some commonly held strengths and needs to some degree, even into the last stage. This makes planning activities a little easier, because activities with the goal of stimulating one or more of these strengths and needs will succeed with most patients. These strengths and needs, along with activities that address them, are listed in Handouts I:10–11 and IV:5–6.

1. Example: Joe is a low second-stage Alzheimer patient. He is physically fit and strong and has the dexterity for large-motor activities. He still loves being outdoors and doing yardwork. He needs to keep using these strengths and long-time interests. Raking leaves and dead grass is a good activity for him. It stimulates strengths he shares with most Alzheimer patients: long-term memory (a habitual skill), large-motor skills, use of strength and dexterity, and all of the senses. It stimulates positive use of perseveration and meets the commonly held need for self-esteem.

2. Most activities provide several types of stimulation. The best activities stimulate several of a person's remaining strengths and meet several needs. For example, social dancing can meet all of the retained strengths and needs on the lists in Handouts IV:5–6.

3. ADLs and IADLs are habitual skills and stimulate all of the commonly held strengths and needs. They should be an integral part of a therapeutic program, in *simplified* form. See activities based on or emphasizing active involvement in ADLs and IADLs in Handouts I:2 and IV:7.

   a. It is often difficult to motivate dementia patients. Motivation for ADLs and IADLs is built in, because patients usually retain some awareness that these are necessary parts of day-to-day life.

   b. Performing ADLs or IADLs increases self-esteem. Performing *simplified* IADLs helps patients feel useful and still connected to daily life.

   c. These activities can easily be incorporated into the program because they must be done anyway.
      • Example: in a small residential care facility, a lettuce and tomato salad is planned for lunch. Under careful supervision and with simple, one-step instructions, residents can prepare the salad. The caregiver can turn a chore that might usually be done *for* residents into an activity *involving* residents.
      • Another example: in a skilled nursing facility, a Halloween party is being planned. With careful planning and simplification of the chores by the activity director, moderately impaired and higher-functioning residents can make all the decorations and refreshments. Simplification is the key (see section III).

E. Patients require a variety of types of stimulation each day.

   1. Anyone feels tired and stiff sitting at a desk all day, or feels tense if he or she is constantly on the run with no time to sit and relax. People need variety. Four basic types of stimulation are needed daily:
      a. large-motor stimulation (e.g., throwing and catching a large ball);
      b. fine-motor stimulation (e.g., folding laundry);
      c. cognitive stimulation (e.g., reminiscing about a favorite vacation or doing a simple crossword puzzle);
      d. social/emotional stimulation (e.g., visiting with children from a neighborhood school).

   2. Large- and fine-motor stimulation are the most successful with dementia patients and should be incorporated into almost all activities.
      a. Active motor activities keep a patient's attention better than passive activity, because these involve several senses plus emotional and cognitive stimulation.

b. Activities that are primarily social or cognitive should involve as much multiple sensory stimulation as possible. For example, if children come to visit, the patients should actively do something with them, not just sit.

III. Adapting activities for use with dementia patients

MODULE IV

A. Read "Planning and Implementing a Therapeutic Activity" (Handout IV:8). These rules also apply for groups but the process becomes more complicated. Members of a group can have widely varying behavior problems, levels of functioning, and interests. (See Module V.)

1. Simplify all activities into very basic steps.
   a. A basic step is an action requiring the retention of only one thought at a time. It does not depend on a previous step or a next step but is complete in itself.
   b. Example: Doing embroidery cannot be divided into single basic, independent steps. Each step of embroidering requires remembering what type of stitch to use, and the stitch itself is complex (it requires the memory of where the previous stitch was taken and a decision on where to place the next one).

2. Higher-functioning patients may still be able to perform activities involving interdependent steps, if the steps are based on the use of *habitual skills* and *long-term memory,* two strengths most dementia patients retain. For example, high-functioning persons may be able to knit, crochet, or embroider if they have done so all their life, but they could *not* learn these skills now.

3. Lower-functioning patients (low second and third stage) can perform only one-step activities repeated over and over (use of the strength of "positive use of perseveration") or may only "rummage" (see Handouts IV:9–10).
   a. Rummaging is random manipulation of objects, with no specific steps. It is a "no-fail" activity. For example, washing dishes involves remembering specific steps that must be performed in order. Moderately impaired patients may enjoy washing or drying only. More severely impaired patients may enjoy just "rummaging," or moving the dishes about in soapy water. They *cannot* actually help wash, but they may enjoy the soothing sensation of movement in the water or the feeling of doing a familiar task.
   b. Rummaging can be successful with all patients. Looking through items that bring back pleasant memories can be successful with high-functioning persons. For example, a high-functioning patient may perceive arranging brightly colored blocks (an activity enjoyed

by lower-functioning patients) as childish but may enjoy looking through a box of old postcards, seashells, or a rock collection.

c. Refer to activities in Handout IV:10.

d. Group exercise: Work in groups of three to plan, explain, and demonstrate an activity for the class. Each group member should have a specific role in the demonstration. Group member 1 explains the project to the class. Group member 2 acts as a caregiver leading the activity. Group member 3 acts the part of a moderately impaired dementia patient with no severe behavior problems (avoid overcomplicating the activity process in this demonstration). While planning the activity, consider:

- How can the activity be simplified into only a few basic steps?
- What are the steps?
- What supplies are needed?
- How should the activity area be arranged?
- Where should supplies be placed?
- How can each step be clearly presented to the patient?

Leading Successful Group Activities; Planning a Day of Activities

MODULE V GOAL Class members will know the basic guidelines for successfully conducting group activities, including adaptations for individual needs and problem behaviors within the activity.

I. Basic rules for choosing and planning therapeutic activities for persons with dementia (also see Module IV)

  A. Activities must be designed to suit the characteristics of each individual patient. They must be designed based on a knowledge of:

    1. the patient's history: social patterns, interests and preferences, physical problems;

    2. the patient's current status, including

      a. severity of neurological symptoms

      b. ability to function in daily life, including emotional state and behavior problems

      c. physical condition.

  B. Activities must be designed to suit the strengths and needs that dementia patients have in common.

    1. Patients need a fairly consistent daily routine of ongoing, simplified, carefully planned therapeutic activity (including rest periods as needed), which maximizes opportunities for success. This helps them

"feel good." It also helps avert unpleasant and difficult situations so common with dementia patients, especially in group settings.

    a. The schedule should also allow for flexibility and spontaneity and should have variety.

    b. *Active* involvement in a variety of large- and fine-motor activities should be emphasized.

2. Individual activities should be divided into a few basic steps. A step is an action based on the retention of one thought at a time and does not depend on a previous thought or action for completion.

    a. Higher-functioning patients may be able to handle several steps.

    b. Lower-functioning patients may need one-step or "no-fail" activities with no specific steps.

3. Patients need to have a pleasant, relaxed environment for activities (see Module III).

4. Patients must experience positive interactions with others during activities. *Always* use the basic rules of positive interaction (Module II).

    a. *Always* remember that patients are adults. Treat them as adults.

    b. Don't rush the patients. Allow plenty of time for activities.

C. Have fun with activities! Be creative. Planning activities and doing them with patients should be enjoyable.

1. Don't be afraid to try new ideas. Experiment with activity ideas from books on activities for dementia patients, adapt activities, get ideas from catalogues of activity supplies, share ideas with other care providers. (See Handout V:1.)

2. Base activities on those commonly enjoyed by cognitively normal older adults. They are familiar, are based on habitual skills, and aid self-esteem. They must be adapted for dementia patients, however.

    a. Many activities can be adapted successfully. Handout V:2 lists activities our centers have adapted for dementia patients.

    b. Remember that activities should have only a few simple independent steps (Handouts V:3–4). Handouts V:5–6 describe a few activities in detail, emphasizing these basic rules.

    c. Many dementia patients can perform very simple activities independently if the staff sets up the activities and helps them begin.

      • Some very simple activities based on positive use of perseveration and which are "no-fail" are listed in Handouts IV:9–10. (Also see Module IV.)

      • Keep in mind that low-functioning patients may have difficulty stopping activities based on positive use of perseveration. This is because stopping is actually an additional step, and they cannot perform it.

3. Care providers should feel confident and comfortable leading activities. Patients can tell if a caregiver is bored or uneasy about an activity and will respond to that.

   a. Example: A care provider who dislikes arts and crafts should not feel obliged to lead a lot of them. If several patients enjoy them, perhaps someone else could plan and lead them, or the caregiver could experiment with very simple, unstructured crafts requiring little advance planning and staff intervention.

   b. Example: If the care provider has a bad headache, perhaps he or she should skip a loud rhythm band or sing-along session and substitute a quieter activity, as long as it is appropriate for the patients.

4. Balance the use of old favorites with new activities. Experimenting is fun and makes the job of caregiving more interesting. Caregivers need to develop enough self-confidence to make a smooth transition to an alternative activity if the experiment flops!

II. Meeting individual needs in the group setting

   A. How can you work with a group of patients and still meet the needs of individuals?

      1. Use small groups. A large group is not usually successful with dementia patients because there are too many different things happening and they are unable to comprehend what is going on. Patients usually do not do well in groups of more than twelve.

      2. Evaluate the full patient group and determine subgroups with common needs and interests. These subgroups can change daily or even during the course of a day. They will change as new patients are added, different behaviors develop, or patients decline.

         a. Before beginning each new activity during the day, always reassess. Activity schedules must be flexible. If preplanned activities do not suit the immediate needs of a patient group, the activity must change. The patients cannot change their behavior to suit the activity.

         b. Subgroups of patients with common interests can be involved in activities based on these common interests. For example, several patients used to play golf. Design a simple golf game. Large-motor activities such as golf will succeed with most patients, and many patients may enjoy a golf game even if golf is not a long-term interest. However, a special golf group and time to reminisce would really benefit those who used to play.

         c. Subgroups of patients with a retained skill in common can be involved in an activity to stimulate this skill. For example, several patients who have high verbal skills can enjoy special reminiscing groups or word games.

    d. Subgroups of patients at the same general level of functioning can be grouped together. For example, several low-functioning patients cannot participate in many of the activities most other patients enjoy. A special table of items to rummage through or sort can be set up for them. Staff members will probably need to stay and keep reengaging them, even in these simple, unstructured tasks.

    e. Subgroups of patients with specific behavior problems or emotional needs should be provided with activities designed to minimize problems and provide a feeling of well-being. For example, several patients are very restless. Their pacing escalates the entire patient group. They should be separated from the other patients and engaged in a vigorous, continuously active, simple large-motor activity such as walking, throwing a ball, raking leaves, sweeping, or wiping off tables. (They would not be able to concentrate on a game in which they had to take turns, such as golf, horseshoes, or a beanbag toss.)

3. Division of the larger patient group into subgroups for activities is called *parallel programing.*

4. What if there are patients who do not seem to fit with any others in a subgroup?

    a. The staff can set aside one or two time periods a day to work with them individually.

    b. Keep experimenting with different groupings and different types of activities to see if they will eventually participate.

    c. Try the activities based on the positive use of perseveration from Handout V:2 and Module IV, which patients can usually perform independently. They may be able to do these by themselves while staff members work with other patients in a group. For example, Mr. Thompson participates only in large-motor group activities such as horseshoes, golf, and ball games. Only two staff members are available, and both are needed for a craft activity with other patients. Mr. Thompson may enjoy looking through a collection of large pictures of various sports or baseball cards, or may enjoy a short sports videotape. Staff members will still need to check on him occasionally to encourage and reengage him in independent activity.

B. Review the general guide to choosing, planning, and implementing group activities (Handout V:3). This guide can be posted on a wall or bulletin board for easy reference when planning activities. Handout V:4 can be used as a quick review.

C. Review activities in Handouts V:5–6. Think about adaptations you would need to make for the involvement of more severely impaired patients or those with disruptive behavior problems.

D. What can the care provider do with residents who won't participate in activities? Read Handout V:7.

III. Planning a day of activities

A. Recreational activities are vital to the therapeutic program. Remember, the goal of the therapeutic program is to keep patients feeling good *all of the time*, to keep them from slipping into difficult behaviors, apathy, or depression. They must be provided with meaningful things to do *whenever* they are needed.

B. How can busy certified nurse assistants (CNAs) or the busy staff of a residential care facility be involved in providing therapeutic activities?

1. Remember that the tasks of daily living are activities, and patients should be involved in them daily (Module IV).
2. The daily schedule should be structured around the provision of *at least* three group activities, freeing staff members for assistance with activities at these times.
3. Provide activities that patients can carry out independently or with little help, so that staff members can perform other duties (the one-step and "no-fail" activities from Module IV and Handout V:2).
4. Staff-to-patient ratios must be higher for therapeutic programing for dementia patients.

C. The use of themes in programing

1. Truly therapeutic programing is fun for care providers and patients alike. Designing and presenting activities based on a common theme throughout the day and over a period of days makes programing more interesting and stimulating for everyone. For example, if the theme is Christmas, patients can make decorations for the Christmas tree each day and then have a tree-decorating party at the end of the week. (They are reminded each day that they will have a tree-decorating party on Friday and that the decorations are for the tree.) Each day a variety of Christmas activities are presented. One day, for example, patients make decorations, sing carols, and make Christmas cookies for the party.
2. The use of themes demands creativity and active involvement in program planning by all staff members.
3. The continuity created by using a theme can stimulate patients' short-term memory and help them clarify time frames.

4. Emphasizing themes on monthly printed calendars adds interest and impresses potential clients.

5. Refer to "Daily and Weekly Themes for Use in Program Planning" (Handout V:8).

D. Planning a schedule of the day

1. Refer to "Schedule of the Day" (Handout V:9), a basic form for scheduling the staff. Support staff for each activity should also be listed. It should help keep staff members from duplicating efforts and avoid staff conflict.

2. The schedule should be fairly consistent from day to day (for instance, meals, an exercise period, and walks could be at the same time each day), but there should be flexibility within the schedule.

3. Allow forty-five minutes to an hour for each activity (patients with short attention spans can wander away and come back). This includes a fifteen-minute transition period. (The actual activity would therefore be between thirty and forty-five minutes long.) Shorter activities are confusing for patients and tiring and stressful for the staff.

4. Offer a variety of types of stimulation each day: large-motor, fine-motor, cognitive, and social/emotional stimulation. Also see Module IV.

5. Alternate types of activities throughout the day. Intensive (harder) activities should follow less-demanding (easier) activities; quiet, more passive activities should follow active ones. For example, follow an active ball game with a more passive sing-along. Follow a word game requiring fairly intense concentration with a walk (less demanding).

   a. Television is usually not a good quiet-time activity.

   b. Most residents cannot follow television and would benefit more from quiet activities that provide more varied types of sensory stimulation.

   • Television distracts when it is on during other activities.

   • Television can dull the residents' remaining ability to respond to other stimuli.

   • Visitors will know that television is being used because it does not require staff involvement. This is not and does not look like therapeutic programing to families and potential clients.

6. Patients are more alert in the morning, so schedule more intensive or new activities then. They are tired in the late afternoon and evening (Sundowner syndrome), so conduct quiet, less-demanding activities then.

7. A simple daily schedule should always be written on the board for patients (for those who can still comprehend it and to orient any fami-

lies or other visitors who may be observing), and it should reflect any current theme.

a. Example: For the Christmas theme mentioned above, the daily schedule should say that the cookies being made are for the tree-decorating party. For the Christmas sing-along, it should say "Christmas sing-along," not just "sing-along."

b. The daily schedule for patient use should always be printed; script is more difficult to read. It should be written in dark ink. Red, yellow, and orange are hard to read from a distance.

c. Higher-functioning patients may use the schedule, at least with added verbal reminders from staff. It adds to their feelings of security, self-esteem, and independence to be able to look at the board to find out what is happening next.

d. The staff must be ready to switch to an alternative activity if patients are restless, tired, etc. *Patients cannot be made to do activities.* The staff must adapt to *their* needs.

Family Dynamics;

Support Systems

for Caregivers

MODULE VI GOAL   Class members will learn more about the necessity for strong support systems in increasing the quality of dementia care, where to go in their community and nationwide for support and networking opportunities, and the importance of fellow staff members and families as part of a strong support system.

I. No one should feel all alone in the job as a care provider.

   A. There are few absolute answers in dementia care. What works with one patient may not work with the next. Each patient can change so rapidly that what works one day may not work the very next. Patients with Alzheimer disease do not improve. Most continue to decline, with death as the final result.

   B. Because professionals as well as families can become discouraged, all care providers must feel they have others they can rely on for support and assistance. They need to develop a support system, a group of people and other resources (agencies, sister facilities, even journals and newsletters) they can count on for information, advice, encouragement, and referrals when things get tough.

   C. Support can come from outside sources such as information and referral agencies and professional journals as well as from other members of one's own professional team.

1. Ongoing support, no matter what the source, is absolutely vital in dementia care and should be carefully cultivated.
2. The care provider must think of *all* available resources as part of the care provider team, working together to provide therapeutic care for each patient. Care providers get discouraged when they are all on their own.
3. See "Effective Support Systems" (Handout VI:1).

II. Professional dementia care information, referral, and assistance resources

A. Good nationwide and community dementia information resources include: Alzheimer disease research and diagnostic centers, resource centers, the Alzheimer's Disease and Related Disorders Association (and other similar organizations), journals, and newsletters (see Handout VI:2).

B. Community long-term dementia care options vary from minimal to full care: from home respite to day care to full-time home care or residential care, then to skilled care and hospice or acute care.

1. Residential and skilled care: care providers need to become familiar with the options in their area.

   a. Residential care does not include medical supervision or services and is not an appropriate placement for patients who need a hgh level of care. It is usually regulated by a state's department responsible for social services. The cost of care is not usually covered by federal or state medical aid programs.

   b. Skilled care facilities are regulated by a state's department responsible for health services and may care for patients with severe, complex medical conditions. They must maintain high standards to care for patients covered by state or federal medical programs. To receive federal Medicare and Medicaid payments, facilities must comply with the Omnibus Budget Reconciliation Act (OBRA) of 1987. These regulations require standardized high-quality care in all skilled nursing facilities providing Medicare and Medicaid coverage nationwide.

   c. Residential and skilled facilities offer many different dementia care options. These can include the following:
      - Special care units for those in different stages or with specific problems, such as units for ambulatory or high-functioning residents and different ones for those with severe behavior problems.
      - Units with different types of security to prevent confused, wandering patients from leaving the facility unattended. Open, alarmed, secured, and locked are common levels of security. If a patient needs secured placement, legal assistance will be required,

but processes vary from state to state. Skilled facilities usually provide more secure placement.

2. Alzheimer family care providers often wish to keep their family member at home, but few dementia-trained home care providers are available. When good home care is available, a combination of home care and day care is often effective.

   a. Families providing home care can get assistance from a hospice in the last stage (also available for patients in residential and skilled care facilities).

   b. Guidelines for the determination of near-death Alzheimer disease are now available. These assist in determining when a hospice can be a care option.

C. Providing families with support

1. Families must plan ahead. Professionals need to be able to provide them with information on different types of health and financial planning and assistance available in their state. These include: living wills, durable power of attorney for finances and health care, conservatorships, ways of protecting assets, Medicare, Medicaid, Supplemental Social Security, long-term care insurance, and where families can go for advice and assistance on these matters.

2. Families need to know where they can go for care advice, referrals, and ongoing support: the local Alzheimer's Disease and Related Disorders Association (or similar organizations), adult day care centers (many offer advice, an opportunity to join a support group, and referrals to any caregiver who calls), mental health agencies, agencies specializing in aging, local support groups.

3. Should professionals give families information on support and long-term care services other than those they provide? For example, if you are an administrator or director of admissions for a residential or skilled care facility, why would you provide families with information on in-home respite and day care? They might decide to use these other resources instead of the services you offer.

   a. Referrals to and networking with other agencies increase your professional standing in the community and can result in increased referrals.

   b. If a care provider presents families with alternative care options and other information on dementia, it shows the family that the primary concern is the welfare of the family and patient.

4. Families of patients need ongoing information and support, even after they place a family member.

   a. Placement can be very difficult for the family, the patient, and the professional staff, since often the families are very concerned about the placement and want to stay involved in patient care decisions.

  b. Families need support from others in similar situations and information from trained professionals. This support assists both the family and the facility working with the family on a regular basis.

III. Understanding and working with the family

A. Families of dementia patients are experiencing the slow death of a family member, which can last for many years. This takes a tremendous toll on families, and many need extensive counseling and support. Professional care providers should refer them to counseling professionals if needed (see Section II).

B. Families often become close to professionals caring for their family member. If professional care providers are knowledgeable about dementia and familiar with the effect it can have on families, they can educate and provide *some* support, but they should *not* take on the role of the mental health or social work professional, unless they are trained in one of those fields.

C. Dealing with families going through such a loss takes compassion, skill, and tact. There are several points that professional care providers should remember:

  1. Know the family well. Know the family's history, the quality of the relationships involved, their feelings about the disease, and their ability to cope. It is necessary to assess the family as well as the patient.

     a. Be aware that families from different ethnic and religious backgrounds may handle aging, the concept of dementia, and the loss of a loved one in very different ways. For example, the ways that an Asian Buddhist family and an Italian Catholic family relate to their family member with dementia and to professional staff may be very dissimilar. These differences must be understood and respected.

     b. The concept of "family" is changing. A care provider may have to work with those who care deeply for the patient but who do not have a traditional relationship to the patient (spouse or child) or who may not even be a "family member" in the traditional sense. (To complicate things further, these people who give care may be from mixed religious and ethnic backgrounds.) Care providers need to be aware of the type of family unit and relationships involved. Read "Nontraditional Families" (Handout VI:3).

  2. Be a good listener. Listen carefully to what a family member is saying, in order to learn more about the family and how they are really feeling.

     a. Often it's necessary to "read between the lines" to determine what the person is trying to say.

b. Sometimes a good listener is all that is needed. With a disease as relentless as Alzheimer and other progressive dementias, sometimes there are no answers, no really useful suggestions.

3. *Always* maintain professional objectivity when dealing with patients' families. Listen and assist *without judging*. The principles listed in "Treating Others Objectively: An Invaluable Skill" (Handout VI:4) should be followed at all times with all family members and patients. They go hand in hand with the positive interaction techniques discussed in Module II.

4. Give advice with great caution. Remember, unless you are highly trained, don't try to act as a professional counselor.

   a. Advice should never sound as if it is the only option. Preface it with, "It might work if . . . " or "Perhaps . . . "

   b. Suggest several options, if possible.

   c. Tell families about trained counseling professionals in the community who might be able to assist them also.

D. Families are not grieving solely for the slow loss of their loved one but are also dealing with other losses as a result of this basic loss. Read "Losses Families May Experience When a Family Member Has Dementia" (Handout VI:5).

E. If family members feel they have experienced many losses due to the patient's disease, they may have more trouble coping with the patient than people who do not feel they are going through as many losses.

1. The *physical burden* is the actual burden—the work—of caring for a dementia patient's physical and behavioral problems and needs.

2. The *emotional burden* is the perceived burden. It is the burden the family member feels due to the physical burden and the other losses he or she has suffered because of the dementing illness. Different caregivers perceive the same amount of physical burden and necessary lifestyle changes in different ways. The emotional burden is based on the quality of the past relationship with the patient, the other losses they feel they have suffered due to the dementia, and the support available from friends and relatives.

3. Families can experience physical and emotional burdens even after engaging professional care for the patient.

4. The "Burden Interview" is a questionnaire useful for measuring a caregiver's emotional burden. It can be found in *The Hidden Victims of Alzheimer's Disease: Families under Stress*, by Orr, Zarit, and Zarit (1985).

5. Refer to the case studies (Handout VI:6).

F. The acceptance of the slow loss of a loved one to dementia can take a long time. Stages of grieving and acceptance have been defined by Kubler-Ross, Kavanaugh, Teusink, Mahler, and others.

1. Family members all go through stages of grief, but not necessarily in the same order. Some people skip stages almost entirely; an event may trigger feelings some thought were resolved; and some never get past a certain stage.

2. Some families finish grieving and let go before the actual death of the family member; some continue to grieve afterward; some may never really stop grieving; and some may go through the stages of grief all over again after the actual death.

3. Five stages that most family members go through are:
   a. *denial* that anything is wrong with the person, perhaps going from doctor to doctor in search of a new diagnosis or treatment;
   b. *overinvolvement,* as they try to help the patient and perhaps slow the disease process once they have acknowledged it;
   c. *anger* that they can't do anything to slow the disease and with all of the losses the family and the person with dementia are experiencing;
   d. *guilt* concerning the anger, unpleasant events in their past relationship with the patient, or decisions that may need to be made for the patient, since he or she can no longer care for himself or herself;
   e. *acceptance,* going on with life.

G. Working with families in different stages of the grieving process.

   1. The first stage, denial. Family members in this stage may resist even basic information on dementia. Quite often, just listening is best at this stage. The professional can provide information whenever family members seem receptive. Providing reading material to take home and look at when they are ready is often good at this point.

   2. The second stage, overinvolvement. Knowledgeable professionals can help family members take action but should watch for harmful, extreme involvement.
      a. A family member very close to the dementia patient, such as a spouse, can have developed a mutual dependency. Caring for the spouse with dementia makes the family member feel needed and wanted.
         • Turning any aspect of care over to others may make the family member feel guilty, weak, or less worthy as a person.
         • The family member needs to be assured that he or she is doing what is best for the patient. For example, if a family member is exhausted with caregiving but refuses to let go, you could say that the family member will be able to do an even better job of

caregiving if he or she gets well, rather than saying that the family member needs to get respite for the sake of his or her own health.

b. Families are usually very receptive to information on dementia and care techniques at this point.

c. If the patient is in a facility, frequent visits and volunteering by the family member may be appropriate.

d. Overinvolvement of family members can be harmful. If it is disturbing to the patient or other residents or if the staff becomes demoralized, encourage less active involvement, such as:
- preparing special projects or treats;
- providing needed materials or supplies;
- helping with a special field trip;
- calling on the telephone.

e. Encourage family members to join a support group to talk things out and share feelings.

3. The third and fourth stages, anger and guilt, respectively. The emotional burden is probably most overwhelming in these stages, because the family member is angry about losses suffered and then feels guilty about these feelings or about steps he or she may have taken (or failed to take) in caring for the patient.

a. Depression is very common among family members in the third and fourth stages. Depressed family members need encouragement to get professional help and to be with other people—support groups and friends and family, away from the patient.

b. What can the professional care provider do for families experiencing guilt and anger?
- Listen.
- Reassure them that these feelings are normal and are shared by other caregivers. Encourage them to join a support group.

c. Care providers must be careful not to take personally the family members' reactions based on anger or guilt.
- Angry family members should never be allowed to verbally abuse the patient or staff but should be handled privately and quietly by appropriate senior staff.
- Family members feeling guilt already feel inadequate. Any suggestions must be carefully worded to show the benefit for the patient. They need reassurance that they are doing what is best for the patient. Reassurances that professional care is of high quality and can provide the patient with the needed stimulation and companionship can help.

4. The fifth stage, acceptance
a. Some family members never reach this final stage; some reach it

and still maintain a special relationship with the patient; others reach it and deliberately avoid any further contact with the patient.

b. Some professionals have difficulty understanding the family member who stops coming to visit a patient or who seems completely indifferent. Again, professionals must be careful not to judge the family member and must put themselves in the family member's shoes. The family member may need to end the relationship to go on with life.

• It is very painful for a family to see a loved one declining so rapidly.

• The patient often acts inappropriately with family members, does not recognize them any more, or at least does not remember them very well. This is one of the most difficult things for many families, and it is easier for some to stop coming to visit than to have a spouse or parent behave so differently or not recognize them any more.

IV. Establishing a productive workplace support system for effective patient care

A. The administrator must establish effective policies and procedures for running an agency or facility, with the goal of establishing the true team environment necessary for therapeutic patient care. Even a small residential care facility needs written policies and procedures.

1. These are written statements that explain to all staff members exactly how the organization is structured and run, its rules and standards, and the criteria for evaluation and advancement.

a. The policies and procedures must change, grow, and evolve with the agency.

b. The staff should know the policies and procedures, should promptly be made aware of any changes, and should know why the changes are being made. Direct care staff should never be the last to know.

2. An administrator should first develop an effective organizational structure, described on an organizational chart, and good job descriptions (see Handouts VI:7–8 for examples). These are the foundations of good policies and procedures. The administrator must evaluate what staff positions are needed and what the exact duties of each position should be. There should be a clear line of supervision, and no employee should have more than one supervisor (unless the tasks required of the position are clearly divided as well).

3. Policies and procedures should carefully present to the staff what is expected of them in the way of professional ethical standards, con-

duct, and dress. Employees must understand that the community's image of an agency or facility depends on how the staff representing the agency present themselves as well as on the appearance and cleanliness of the building and, of course, on the quality of care. Read "Employees with Pride in Their Profession" (Handout VI:9).

4. Procedures for hiring, training, evaluating, promoting, and terminating staff members must be carefully developed.

5. Patient care policies must be in writing, even in small residential care facilities and by home care agencies. These should include emergency measures, admission and discharge criteria, procedures for storing and dispensing medication, etc.

6. There are many books and courses on writing policies and managing personnel, and consultants can be hired to help establish and write policies and procedures.

B. How can an administrator choose the right people for the vitally important job of providing direct patient care?

1. The supervisor should write down the personal qualities required and the exact duties of the position. These are the basis for the job description. See Handout VI:8.

2. How can a supervisor tell if a person being interviewed is right for the job?

   a. The administrator or immediate supervisor should compose a list of relevant questions and ask all applicants the same questions.

   b. The supervisor should observe the applicant in actual patient interactions.

C. A new employee must know the exact duties and receive proper training.

1. Training new staff members takes time. New, untrained staff members are often put with patients simply because they are desperately needed.

   a. The supervisor should try to have experienced staff members cover the position until new staff members have completed comprehensive dementia care training. Or, after the new staff person has had some basic training, the supervisor should pair him or her with an experienced staff member—a mentor—until the formal dementia care training is complete.

   b. The supervisor should continue using the mentor system until he or she is sure of the new staff person's performance on the job.

2. The supervisor should keep all employees informed of their performance on a regular basis. This is especially important with new employees. Praise and prompt resolution of problems should take place regularly.

D. The supervisor should try to keep morale high and encourage teamwork and mutual support among the patient care staff. Staff members should be encouraged to communicate job-related problems to their supervisor. They should be included in decision making.

1. Teamwork and good communication increase staff morale and self-esteem.

2. Teamwork and good communication are essential in work with dementia patients, because behavior management requires a consistent approach by *all* staff members and behavior problems can be managed only if all staff people work together in solving them.

3. Hold weekly staff meetings and encourage staff members to talk informally daily. Staff meetings are a good time to try to strengthen mutual support systems among team members. In staff meetings, the supervisor should:

   a. guide and participate in, but never dominate, the discussion;
   b. not separate himself or herself from the group by sitting behind a desk;
   c. really listen;
   d. act on suggestions;
   e. encourage discussion and team planning of patient care and behavior-management strategies, thus making direct care staff members feel that they are a vital part of the patient care team;
   f. keep the staff informed of important administrative news; show them their intelligence and opinions are respected.

4. The supervisor should stress the importance of the job of the direct care staff and show pride in the facility or agency and in each staff person's work.

5. The supervisor should "be there," observe, listen, talk, assist, and work with them on the job occasionally. Supervisors distance themselves from their staff if they never join staff members in the actual performance of their duties. The staff then feel that the supervisor does not understand or respect their work.

6. The supervisor should be lavish with genuine praise, but should not praise unless it is really deserved.

7. The supervisor should resolve job performance problems quickly and completely by:

   a. always giving criticisms and suggestions privately;
   b. always starting with the positive;
   c. making "I think" or "I feel" statements and using suggestions such as "Could you . . . ?" or "Co you think we could . . . ?" rather than orders such as "You must" or "You cannot";

d. giving the employee time to respond, then really listening and thinking about the responses;

e. documenting serious problems in case termination becomes necessary—always making sure that this is stated in written policy and that employees know the procedure when they start work;

f. continuing to monitor problem employees, quickly praising improvements in job performance and talking over any new problems;

g. being consistent: not noting performance problems in one employee while ignoring them in another.

8. An agency or facility should provide "perks" like staff parties, special lunches, even an extra-long break once in a while. Little things such as a place to store belongings, an engraved name tag, or a change in position title can mean a lot to staff members.

9. There should be opportunities for advancement. An agency or facility should do the following:

a. Have written policies on how advancement, raises, or bonuses are awarded. Make sure the staff knows what they are. Give higher raises or bonuses for exceptional performance. Be objective and consistent in any awards.

b. Consider bonuses, "comp time," extra training opportunities, or extra vacation days for staff members who perform exceptionally, act as a trainer or mentor for a new staff member, or get extra training or a degree on their own. Keep a written record of all exceptional performance, note it in evaluations, and consider it when opportunities for advancement become available.

c. Not put off raises or advancement unless it is absolutely necessary due to financial cutbacks. A good staff is a facility or agency's best asset.

V. Managing stress

A. What is stress? It is basically a feeling that there is too much to manage, do, or decide adequately. Tension, strain, unhappiness, or discontent with day-to-day life can develop as a result.

B. The first step in stress management is deciding when the stress is too much. Some stress is healthy. Being busy and involved makes life seem worthwhile, but each person handles stress differently.

C. If a person is "burning out," stress has reached an unmanageable level. The person cannot cope or give any more. Signs of burnout are:

1. *Physical symptoms:* tiring more easily; complaints such as headaches, aches and pains, a lingering cold; not "looking good."

2. *Emotional symptoms:* feeling cynical or disillusioned; unexplained sadness; visiting and talking with friends less frequently; inability to laugh and joke about oneself; feeling that sex is "too much trouble"; increased irritability; loss of interest in activities previously enjoyed.

3. *Work performance problems:* working harder and enjoying it less; forgetting appointments and possessions; feeling too busy to finish routine tasks; feeling lost or disoriented when the work day is at an end; inability to set priorities.

D. If a person feels that he or she is burning out, the person should try to determine the cause of the feelings. Are they related to work or to home life? If the stress is a combination of things, the person should try to isolate the primary stressor.

1. If the stress originates at home, it is essential to try to forget it at work. Simply realizing that a stressor from home is affecting work may make it easier to keep the two separate.

2. To reduce or eliminate a stressor, a person must plan carefully. One symptom of stress is reduced ability to think through and complete tasks, so this may be difficult. The person must:
   a. isolate the cause, or the primary cause, of the stress;
   b. figure out a way or ways to try to change the situation and write them down;
   c. take time to try to work toward a solution, then give one possible solution a good try before trying another.

3. The stress style test and relaxation suggestions in Handouts VI:10–11 may be useful in understanding, measuring, and relieving stress and burnout.

E. The management of stress is especially important when working with dementia patients, since they will respond negatively to signs of stress in the caregiver. However, caregiving itself can cause excessive stress—it is emotionally exhausting!

1. It is vital that a professional *never* let stress affect the treatment of patients.

2. The care provider can let out anger or hostility by exercising vigorously, talking with a friend, or using relaxation techniques, but *never* by acting inappropriately with patients.

3. Patients with dementia are very vulnerable, because the care of *all* of their needs is in a caregiver's hands.

4. Even when caregivers think they are in control and hiding stress, patients will react to subtle tension or anger. Remember, persons with dementia must be treated in a consistently positive, calm, accepting

manner or they will become increasingly anxious and catastrophic reactions can develop.

F. Administrators must be aware of stress reactions in employees and do everything they can to make the workplace a positive one—to keep work from being a cause of excessive stress. The self-esteem and morale of the staff are essential to the success of a facility or an agency. With morale and self-esteem low, teamwork and mutual support systems crumble.

G. "Food for thought": If professionals find patient care stressful, think how family care providers feel.

H. Refer to the body scan exercise (Handout VI:12). It is a good way to reduce stress in the middle or at the end of a busy day—and a good way to refresh oneself for the important job of providing the very best therapeutic program possible!

HANDOUTS

Normal Physical Changes and Common Conditions and Diseases of Aging

All the following bodily systems slowly decline in efficiency with age, but don't despair! Normally functioning older adults can do an amazing job of compensating for these changes (*active aging*), and most continue to live long, continuously productive lives.

Skin dries, thins, wrinkles, and sags, and sweat glands become less efficient.
   CONDITIONS AND DISEASES: Skin can easily tear. Skin cancer is more common.

Bones become brittle.
   CONDITIONS AND DISEASES: Fractures can occur more easily. Osteoporosis and osteoarthritis are common.

Muscle mass is reduced. The body has an increased fat-to-lean body mass ratio. The body is not as firm, and muscle strength is weakened.
   CONDITIONS: Stooped posture and slower gait are common.

The *urinary tract* becomes less efficient. Kidneys have decreased function and increased numbers of abnormal blood clusters.
   CONDITIONS AND DISEASES: The prostate frequently enlarges in men. Frequent urination and difficulty urinating are common problems, and kidney infections, kidney failure, and prostate cancer are more common.

Lungs have decreased elasticity and movement.
   CONDITIONS AND DISEASES: Lung capacity and endurance may greatly decrease, and the chance of respiratory illness increases.

The *cardiovascular system* becomes less efficient. Arteries elongate and thicken, and the heart rate decreases. Heart valve tissue hardens.

CONDITIONS AND DISEASES: Blood circulation and endurance may be slowed. Heart disease, heart failure, hardening of the arteries, high blood pressure, and strokes are more common.

The *immune system* is less efficient. The body has a reduced ability to fight off diseases and to recover from illnesses.

CONDITIONS AND DISEASES: A person may suffer from more minor and major illnesses and be ill for longer periods of time.

The *nervous system* loses efficiency due to decreased brain weight and cortical cell count. This is benign forgetfulness.

DISEASES: Diseases such as Parkinson and Alzheimer disease occur.

The *intestinal tract* contains an increased number of abnormal blood vessels, and peristalsis is slowed.

CONDITIONS AND DISEASES: Impactions and hemorrhoids can occur, and colon cancer is more common.

Hearing is reduced due to degenerative changes such as obstruction in the eustachian tubes and loss of auditory neurons. Hearing declines in almost all older people.

CONDITIONS: Severe hearing loss, especially for high frequencies, is common.

Vision is poorer, due to decreased pupil size, growth of the lens, and fatty deposits in the eye. Difficulty with near vision is almost universal.

CONDITIONS AND DISEASES: A white ring around the eye often appears due to fatty deposits. Colors can appear more yellow due to the thickening of the lens. Poorer vision under darkened conditions, poorer judgment of distance, and increased sensitivity to glare can occur. Cataracts and glaucoma are common.

The *sense of smell* probably declines. Research is limited.

CONDITIONS: Significant loss of this sense affects taste, increases difficulty distinguishing between similar foods, and may result in a reduction in food intake and loss of weight.

The *sense of touch* probably declines with poor circulation and with decreased use, but little research has been done.

CONDITIONS: Reduced ability to distinguish between similar objects, textures, and hot and cold could result.

The *sense of taste* declines due to poorer taste buds, decreased saliva flow, and poorer teeth and gums.

CONDITIONS AND DISEASES: Enjoyment of food can be reduced. Weight loss can occur. Gum diseases are more common.

The Activities of Daily Living (ADLs) and Instrumental Activities of Daily Living (IADLs)

The Activities of Daily Living (ADLs) are the most basic activities of day-to-day life. They are fundamental necessities and must be done daily or even several times daily for the maintenance of good health. Therefore, a person who needs even minimal help with such basic activities usually cannot live alone. These activities are:

eating;

transferring in and out of bed, chairs, etc., without assistance;

mobility: walking inside and out without assistance from another person (may use a cane or walker);

dressing;

grooming: brushing teeth and hair, shaving, applying makeup;

bathing;

toileting;

continence care.

The Instrumental Activities of Daily Living (IADLs) are generally more complex and less routine in nature than the ADLs. Persons who cannot perform these activities but can still manage the ADLs often do not need constant monitoring. They do not need help from others as frequently or for such long periods as those who cannot perform the ADLs. Therefore, they may still be able to live alone, with part-time assistance from others. These activities are:

shopping;

meal preparation;

housework;

laundry;

taking public transportation;

using the telephone;

taking medications;

money management.

Alzheimer Disease and Other Causes
of Dementia: An Overview

Alzheimer disease is a neurological disorder that destroys certain vital cells of the brain and produces intellectual disability (dementia). It was described in 1907 by Dr. Alois Alzheimer, a German neurologist, who noted that the gray matter of the outer layer (cortex) of the brain, where thought processes evolve, was degenerated and destroyed in his patients suffering from presenile (before sixty-five) or senile (after sixty-five) dementia. These nerve cells can now be shown by electron microscopy to have within them abnormal rigid structures, called tangles, which are composed of numerous groups of paired, twisted, silk-like filaments. Next to these degenerating nerve cells, plaques containing an abnormal protein called amyloid can be seen. The walls of numerous cerebral blood vessels also show deposits of amyloid protein.

Symptoms

The result of this damage to the brain produces slow and insidious symptoms, with the earliest impairment being that of recent memory. Soon simple, everyday chores (e.g., driving an automobile or dressing) become increasingly difficult. As the disease progresses, memory loss increases, reasoning deteriorates, concentration degenerates along with speech and handwriting, and personality may change. Placid persons may become violent; active persons may become placid and inert. With progressive deterioration comes a disorientation of person (e.g., confusion of a spouse with a parent, or disorientation to time and place). In addition, behavior problems become marked (e.g., wandering and getting lost, the inability to start and complete a task successfully, or repeatedly asking the same question because of recent memory loss). Gradual losses occur in the ability to communicate and understand the spoken or written word. Incontinence, depressed reflexes, and similar neurological abnormalities may also appear at this stage. Psychotic symptoms such as delusions, hallucinations, paranoid ideation, and severe agitation may also become apparent. In the final stages of the disease, patients may be totally unable to care for themselves. The immediate cause of death is often pneumonia or other infections that the Alzheimer patient can't fight due to his or her debilitated condition. No treatment is known to reverse this unrelenting process, although treatment of some behavioral symptoms may be successful.

Relationship to Down syndrome

Down syndrome individuals over the age of forty invariably have the same lesions as in Alzheimer disease, and a large number of these individuals become demented. Recent research has shown that the amyloid present in the cerebral vessels and plaques in Alzheimer disease and Down syndrome are composed of a unique protein called the beta protein. This protein is coded for by a gene on chromosome 21 (the Down syndrome chromosome), and this indicates that Down syndrome is clearly linked in pathology to Alzheimer disease.

Statistics

Alzheimer disease is age-related but is not caused by aging, as are a number of other disease processes (e.g., diabetes, arthritis, osteoporosis). In the United States, according to the National Institute on Aging's *Progress Report on Alzheimer's Disease, 1993* (NIH Publication No. 93-3409):

Over 4 million adults are affected, at a cost for care of over $90 billion annually. This cost is greater than for the care of heart disease, cancer, and stroke combined.

One out of six people over age sixty-five is affected.

It is the fourth most common cause of death. One family in three will see one of the parents succumb to this disease.

Each year, 120,000 people die from it.

Alzheimer disease is responsible for over 50 percent of nursing home admissions.

$90 billion is spent per year on medical bills, nursing home costs, and lost productivity.

Diagnosis

Secondary dementias: The diagnosis of Alzheimer disease is best made by an experienced physician in conjunction with a multidisciplinary team who must rule out other diseases. Some usually treatable (potentially reversible or non-progressive) causes of memory loss are secondary dementias (other symptoms are also present). These account for 20 percent of those with dementia, and some are:

alcoholism (severe: Korsakoff syndrome);

barbiturate intoxication;

multiple drug administration;

vitamin B_{12} deficiency;

potassium loss from self-purgation;

poor nutrition;

metabolic disorders (e.g., Addison disease);

cerebral diseases (e.g., slow-growing tumors, multiple cerebral emboli);

infections;

psychiatrically treatable depression (a pseudo or "false" dementia).

Extensive chemical, physical, neurological, and psychiatric tests must be performed to eliminate curable / treatable conditions.

Primary dementias: The vast majority of dementias (80 percent) are designated as primary dementias. Dementia is the primary symptom, and primary dementias are caused by degenerative diseases that are either untreatable or rarely treatable (they are irreversible and progressive). Multi-infarct dementia caused by hypertension or diabetes is a possible exception to this, since the control of the diseases by medication may eliminate the progression of dementia. According to G. G. Glenner, "Alzheimer's Disease," *Encyclopedia of Human Biology* (New York: Academic Press, 1994), 1:103–11, causes of primary dementia and frequency of occurrence (incidence at autopsy) are:

Alzheimer disease	62.6%
multi-infarct dementia	21.4%
mixed Alzheimer disease and multi-infarct dementia	6.3%
Pick disease	3.0%
Creutzfeldt-Jacob and "other"	< 1.0%
Parkinson disease	5.7%

Treatment

Until the nature of the Alzheimer disease process is discovered, treatment must be directed at the symptoms. No proven curative treatment is yet available, although medication may be appropriate in some cases for the treatment of behavior problems. Also, involvement in a positive activity program may keep the victim functioning at the highest level possible. Education of the public in understanding the disease and the elimination of fear and fantasy about Alzheimer disease is vital. Developing support and respite for the family caregiver who provides the majority of care (the secondary victim) and making available long-term care in appropriate facilities are equally as important.

Genetic Risk

Genetic researcher Dr. Leonard Heston, while at the University of Washington, Seattle, clarified some risk questions based on his research. Given a *proven* case of Alzheimer disease, there is a risk of 33 to 50 percent that a second case may appear in that family. The earlier the onset of illness in a given case, the higher the risk for other family members. This risk ranges from near 50 percent in families with onset before age forty-five to about the same as the general population if onset is over age seventy. These risks are age-specific and *must* be cited as such (e.g., when a family member has an onset at age fifty-five, first-degree relatives have a risk of 5 percent at age sixty-five, 14 percent at age seventy-five, and 23 percent at age eighty-five). (First-degree relatives are brothers, sisters, parents, and children of a patient.)

Dr. Heston's statement emphasizes some things that appear to affect the percentage of risk:

A previous *proven* case in the family increases risk. This means autopsy-confirmed diagnosis of a family member in the past.

Possible risk factors vary widely, based on
- other proven cases in the family
- the age of onset of proven case(s)
- the age of those for whom the risk is being computed.

Additional genetic research is also being done on chromosomes 1, 14, 19 (Apolipoprotein), as well as on chromosome 21.

Conclusion

There are many challenges facing researchers, governmental and private providers of health care, family and professional caregivers, and the population in general. Discovering diagnostic tools, causes, and treatments for Alzheimer disease must proceed as health care providers and families work on means of caring for all the primary and secondary victims of this devastating disease.

The Pathogenesis of Alzheimer Disease

The beta protein precursor (a larger "parent" protein) is taken up by cerebro-vascular endothelial cells. It is then cleaved to form amyloid fibers (1).

The amyloid breaks the blood-brain barrier (2) in arterioles and binds to brain cell (neuron) membranes. It then forms abnormal neurofilaments (paired helical filaments), which cause the death of the cell (3).

Amyloid seepage through the arteriole walls also produces the amyloid cores of neuritic plaques (4).

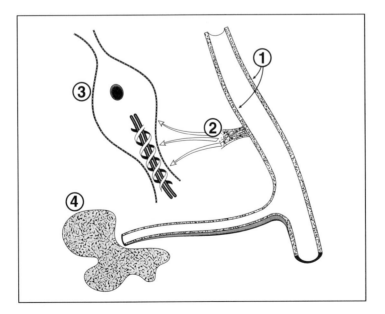

Illustration of CAT Scans

The difference between normal aging, Alzheimer disease, and multi-infarct dementia in the brain is illustrated in these three diagrams. Cerebral atrophy with extensive loss of gray matter characterizes Alzheimer disease, while both gray matter and white matter are involved in multi-infarct dementia.

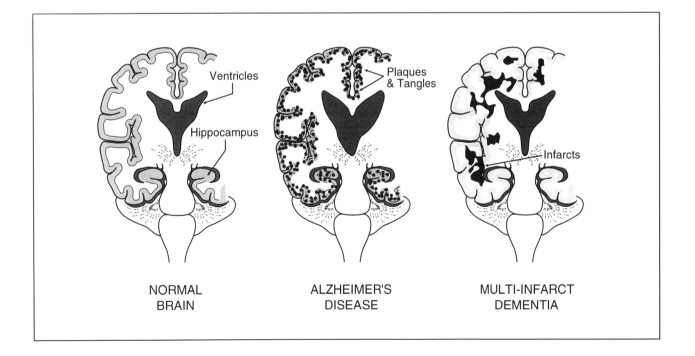

Common Neurological Symptoms of Dementia

These symptoms are evident to some degree in even the earliest stages of dementia and are eventually *universal.* All patients will decline in all areas as the dementia increases; however, patients will *not* decline in each problem area at the same rate.

Plan a program for patients which helps them use their strongest skills as much as possible. Avoid activities that require the use of very weak skills.

Remember, use the three stages of dementia only as general guidelines. Patients may be able to function better in some areas than in others.

Neurological functions that decline as dementia progresses are:

Perception (interpreting sensory cues—interpreting relationships between objects and self and environment); *and* Organization of movement (using objects correctly)

Attention span and concentration

Language (expressive, receptive)

Memory (awareness, retention, retrieval)

Appropriate emotional reaction and appropriate degree of reaction

Abstract reasoning *and* Judgment—thinking (following sequences, forming concepts, reaching conclusions)

Memory Trigger: Common Neurological Symptoms of Dementia

The following word association cue may help you remember the six common neurological symptoms of Alzheimer disease and related dementia. Spell out Mr. Palmer's name. Each letter is the first letter of a symptom. (You will need to remember that the first and last letters of "Palmer" stand for two related symptoms each.)

"Mr. Palmer has Alzheimer disease." He has problems with:

P erception *and* Organization of movement

A ttention span

L anguage

M emory

E motional control

R easoning *and* Judgment

The Three Stages of Irreversible and Progressive Dementia

Stage One: Onset

Often this stage is deceptive, with:

Recent memory loss and mild aphasia

Confusion, decreased concentration

Impaired judgment and increased anxiety

Personality change (e.g., depression)

Progressive loss of intellectual abilities, verbal expression (aphasia), reading (alexia), writing (agraphia), sensory powers (agnosia)

Stage Two: Middle

All symptoms of Stage One are increased:

Restlessness and agitation

Perseveration (persistence of one idea or one answer)

May become lost

Excessive skeletal muscle tone with unsteady gait and stiffness (hypertonia)

Confusion: toileting and continence care

Stage Three: Terminal

Needs constant supervision and assistance

Delusions and hallucinations

Incontinence: urinary, then fecal

Difficulty in swallowing (choking and aspiration)

Emaciation

Loss of responsiveness

Case Studies: Symptoms, Strengths, and Needs

The following case studies illustrate common neurological symptoms, remaining strengths, and needs of persons with dementia; how these symptoms are manifested in the three stages of the disease; and excess disability.

Warren

HISTORY. Warren is a fairly young Alzheimer patient. He was diagnosed about a year and a half ago. He is sixty-eight years old, extremely fit and handsome, and continues to dress well. His dementia is progressing quite rapidly.

He graduated from college in California and owned and operated bookstores north of Los Angeles for many years. Soon after Warren retired (two years ago), his wife died. Warren started to show signs of memory loss and reduced interest and involvement in the activities of daily life before her death, but his son and wife thought he was simply having trouble adapting to retirement. After her death, the son was still not sure that anything was really wrong. He thought the symptoms might be those most people would exhibit after the death of a spouse. Because the symptoms did not go away, however, Warren was eventually evaluated by a neurologist and was diagnosed with Alzheimer disease.

Warren moved in with his son, daughter-in-law, and their two small children eight months ago. He began attending day care three days a week six months ago. In some areas, his functions remain quite high; in others, they are severely impaired.

CURRENT ABILITY TO FUNCTION. It is difficult for the casual observer to tell that anything is wrong with Warren because he looks intelligent and fit and acts in socially appropriate ways. He understands conversation well (receptive language), has better short-term memory than many other high-functioning patients, and seems to retain more complex thought patterns and the ability to form concepts. He retains the capacity to perform complex large-motor activities, such as bowling, shuffleboard, and horseshoes. He can follow verbal instructions and visual cues (short-term memory, concept formation, sequencing, and visual perception) for these large-motor activities. His attention span is very good. He does not seem to have excessive emotional swings and is rarely upset or angry.

Warren's expressive language ability is very poor. However, his receptive ability seems better. He understands conversation and grasps some concepts so well that he is frustrated when he cannot respond adequately. Staff members adapt to this disability by continuing to speak to him about more complex ideas, while making sure he can reply using very simple sentences. The staff would be encouraging an excess disability if they did not continue to encourage him to use his good short- and long-term memory, thought processes, and receptive language ability.

Warren also has great difficulty with less familiar fine-motor tasks. His perception in fine-motor activities such as cutting, gluing, and painting in unfamiliar craft activities is very poor. He usually gets up and walks away from them. Again, he does not get very angry, but the staff can tell he is upset. In cooking projects he can grate cheese and stir. He seems to enjoy these activities, because they are very familiar habitual skills based in long-term memory.

Warren's self-esteem is very fragile. He seems to grasp when activities have been deliberately simplified for him and will then not participate. He will not participate in very complex activities either, however, since he seems to know he will have difficulty (concept formation). He sits alone in the living room at these times, but he can still take the initiative and pick up a magazine or occasionally engage someone in simple conversation.

SUMMARY. Warren appears to be primarily in Stage One of Alzheimer disease. His short-term memory, thought processes, receptive language ability, social skills, and large-motor skills remain at a very high level. His needs to maintain his self-esteem and to engage in meaningful conversation with others are very high and are reinforced by the staff. Warren's fine-motor perceptual abilities and expressive language ability are more at a Stage Two level. He knows he has problems in these areas and avoids situations requiring him to use these skills.

Madeline

HISTORY. Madeline is a fairly healthy, active Alzheimer patient in her early seventies. Her only physical problems are severe myopia (nearsightedness), which she has had since childhood, and mild obesity. She was diagnosed with Alzheimer disease eight years ago and is declining at a moderate rate.

Madeline had a high school education and was trained as a secretary. She was married for many years and raised five children. After a divorce in her late fifties, she lived by herself and worked as a secretary. In her last two years at work, employers began to notice a decline in her general performance. She was discharged with medical disability.

Madeline's children all live out of state and have a great deal of difficulty understanding and coping with her disability. For that reason, Madeline moved in with a younger sister when she could not care for her needs alone in her apartment.

As the disease progressed, the sister could no longer care for Madeline, so placed her in a small residential care facility for Alzheimer patients. However, the facility also had difficulty managing her behaviors, and she was soon moved to a special care Alzheimer unit of a skilled nursing facility.

CURRENT ABILITY TO FUNCTION. Madeline's disability is now quite severe, and she has been diagnosed as generally in the very late second or early third stage of Alzheimer disease. She has lost most of her long- and short-term memory and cannot engage in meaningful conversation, though she does understand simple one-step instructions for some fine- and large-motor tasks very well. She does not act in socially appropriate ways. She sometimes smiles at staff but is not animated. She sometimes seems a little angry or sad but does not express these emotions actively. She exhibits many types of perseveration. She walks to the bathroom in her room or the one next to the activity room, seats herself, flushes the toilet, and washes her hands over and over each day. In addition, she almost constantly rocks back and forth and exhibits tardive dyskinesia (tongue thrust). She also repeats the same phrases over and over. Other patients are aware of these behaviors and are irritated by them. Several patients become angry if she is near them. Nursing and/or activity staff members must be constantly near Madeline to steer her away from these contacts and also to distract her from her many trips to the bathroom. Madeline does not appear to be aware of the reactions of the other patients.

Problems with eating have occurred recently, and she needs constant monitoring. She can manage food with utensils well and has a large appetite (a concern because of her tendency to be overweight). However, she often does not swallow and will keep putting bites of food in her mouth without chewing. She continues to rock back and forth while she eats. She can no longer participate in any food-preparation activities designed by the activity department and must be closely watched in craft activities, since she will eat ingredients and try to drink the paint and glue.

Even though Madeline has many problems, she does not function poorly in all areas. Her perceptual and organization of movement abilities in some familiar fine- and large-motor activities appear to be almost at the Stage One level. If she is wearing her glasses, the activity staff can easily motivate her to cut out complex fabric and paper designs, and she can do fairly complex jigsaw puzzles that few other patients are able to complete. She has good balance and coordination in exercise and familiar large-motor games, but the activity staff must be there constantly to reengage her, since her attention span is very short. If nurse assistants give her one-step instructions and continually reengage her, she can dress herself, including buttoning blouses and tying shoes.

She will clear the activity room table after craft or food preparation activities, clean it, and even wash dishes at the activity room sink with some reminders. She used to play the piano and can still pick out bits and pieces of favorite tunes. These are habitual skills based on basic large- and fine-motor functions.

Madeline needs her glasses to perform almost all activities, and all staff members check to make sure she is wearing them. If she is not, she has much more difficulty moving about and doing things. Her awareness of her surroundings greatly decreases, and she simply spends her day pacing the center. If her glasses are not on, an excess disability is created (a disability in excess of what is actually caused by the dementia).

SUMMARY. Madeline is approaching Stage Three of Alzheimer disease. Her memory, expressive language ability, attention span, concentration, abstract reasoning, and judgment are all severely impaired. However, she retains good perceptual skills, evident in her ability to perform tasks based on habitual skills. She has kept other strengths, such as basic large- and fine-motor functions, positive use of perseveration, and the basic senses, and still has all the basic needs, to a reduced extent. She has lost other skills that are usually retained into the last stage, including most of her long-term memory and her ability to express emotion. Although she uses perseveration positively, she also has severe behavior problems associated with perseveration.

Strengths Commonly Retained by Persons with Dementia

Unless other physical problems interfere, most of these strengths are retained into the final stage of dementia. Activities requiring the use of these strengths are the best type for dementia patients.

Strengths that are retained or decline very gradually:

Habitual skills:
Social
Any task performed repetitively throughout life

Remote memory:
Memories of past achievements, old friends, special events, etc.

Basic large- and fine-motor functions:
Strength
Dexterity
Muscle control
Balance

The basic senses:
Vision
Hearing
Taste
Touch
Smell
Rhythm
Movement

Emotion:

    Redirection of negative emotions

    Active expression of positive emotion

Positive use of perseveration:

    Persistence in repetition of enjoyable one- or two-step tasks

HANDOUT I:10

Psychosocial Stimulation Needs Commonly Retained by Persons with Dementia

After one's basic physical needs are met, feeling good about oneself and about life depends on the quality of interactions with other human beings. Even though they often cannot express the need for or initiate positive interactions with others, Alzheimer patients continue to retain the need for psychosocial stimulation. These needs may even increase as memory loss, loss of communication skills, confusion, anxiety, and disorientation caused by the dementing illness increase.

Patients continue to need the following:

A sense of security:
  A calm, predictable environment
  Acceptance by others

Self-Esteem:
  Maintenance of some control over one's environment
  Maintenance of some control over affairs and one's self
  Confidence in ability to continue to perform useful tasks

Inclusion in a group:
  Meaningful communication (verbal and nonverbal)
  Active participation in the group

Behavior-Rating Instrument

BEHAVIORAL RATING INSTRUMENT

Patient Name: William Bentley   **Date of Rating**

LIGHT STAGE:
* Feeds self with minimal assistance
__Dresses self appropriately 80-90% of the time
* Occasional daytime incontinence (1 to 2 times a month)
* Needs no assistance with toileting 80-90% of the time (may need reminder)
* Can handle small amounts of money; needs help with larger transactions
* Can perform some household tasks (meal preparation, gardening, laundry, repairs, "housework," shopping, talking on telephone)
* Occasional loss of orientation to place, especially in less familiar settings; occasionally gets lost out-of-doors (25% of the time)
__Has some anxiety and/or depression
* Has some personality change

MODERATE STAGE:
__Needs assistance with eating or can feed self modified food
* Uses wrong sequence when dressing self, commonly forgets items (40-50% of the time)
__Daytime incontinence (1 to 2 times a week)
__Needs some assistance with toileting and needs reminding
__Requires assistance in handling money
__Has difficulty performing household tasks
__Some loss of orientation to time, place, and familiar people; can find way about indoors 50% of the time
* May show restless, confused agitation or withdrawn behavior; tends to pace
__May be angered easily and may be combative
__Able to communicate needs, though with difficulty, and perhaps in garbled speech or incomplete sentences
__Tends to wander out

SEVERE STAGE:
__Has to be fed
__Unable to dress self
__Incontinent of urine; may have fecal incontinence
__Requires assistance with toileting
__Unable to handle money
__Unable to perform household tasks
__Disoriented to time and place and familiar people; generally unaware of surroundings, year, season
__May be agitated, exhibits repetitive behavior
__May exhibit (previously non-existent) violent behavior
__May continually repeat words, syllables, or sounds, sometimes loudly in disruptive manner, or may be non-responsive
__May be destructive of one's environment, including one's clothing or self
__Has little or no ability to communicate one's needs verbally
__May wander out unless watched at all times

<u>Source:</u> Form from State of California, Department of Aging. Sacramento, Calif.

Physician's Report

```
                         PHYSICIAN'S REPORT
NOTE TO PHYSICIAN:
     The person whose name appears below is an applicant for a
licensed day care program.  This facility provides the personal
care and supervision normally provided by a relative to a member of
the family.  A current health report is required.

Name and  William Hayes Bentley            Date of exam: 1/2/96
address:  1330 Wedgewood Way, Apt. 321     Date of birth 7/6/1914
          San Diego, CA  92073             Sex  Male
Length of time under your care:  1 year
PRIMARY DIAGNOSIS:  Probable early Alzheimer disease


  SECONDARY DIAGNOSIS: Depression    occasional angina
                       osteoarthritis    cataract left eye
  TUBERCULOSIS CLEARANCE: negative 1/2/96
              Date of last negative chest x-ray (within 1 yr)
                        1/2/96
              Date of last negative skin test (within 1 yr)
HEALTH HISTORY:
     Past illness, medical treatments, hospitalizations:
                     Left hip replacement-3/88

     History of present illness: Symptoms of AD within past year
       Difficulty driving, grooming, cleaning for past year.  Neurological
       exam 6/95 (Dr. B. Hayes)             Diagnosis: probable AD
     Current Medications: Cardizem: 30mg 4x/daily
                          Ibuprofen: 200mg 2 or 3u/daily

     Allergies: None


PHYSICAL ASSESSMENT:
     General appearance: Somewhat obese
     Integument:  None
     Head, eyes, ears:   cataract: vision gradually deteriorating
     Nose:   no problem
     Mouth, throat:  "
     Respiratory:  "
     Cardiovascular: occasional angina
     Gastrointestinal:  no problem
     Genitourinary:  "
     Musculoskeletal:  calcification of some joints
     Neurological: probable Alzheimer; depression



_____     Name  J.T. Newman, MD, Suite 200
Signature                           Address 200 North Drive, SD, CA 92035
                                    Phone No. (619) 436-1866
Date:    1/2/96
```

Patient Profile and Social History

PATIENT PROFILE AND SOCIAL HISTORY

NAME__William Hayes Bentley_____
AGE___82____
BIRTH DATE___7/6/1914_____

MEDICAL INFORMATION
Mobility: ambulatory___*____ walker_____ cane_____wheelchair_____
Vision: normal_rt. eye_ normal w/ glasses_____ poor_lt. eye_blind____
Hearing: normal__*___ impaired_____ deaf_____ hearing aid_____
Hand Dominance __left_____ Special Diet __N/A_____

BACKGROUND
Living Arrangement__apartment alone since wife's death: 1982____
Local Family Support__one or two friends, son in L.A._____
Level of Education_1 year college_ Languages Spoken_English_____
Former Occupation_Armstrong Tile Sales____
Other Skills_printer after college, woodworking for neighbors____
_____
Other jobs held_worked in sales at several companies, printer___
Place of Birth_Indianapolis, IN__ Siblings_1 sister in Wisc., 1 brother died:1981
Marital Status M___ W_*_ D___ Sp___ Sg___ Length of Time_41 years_
No. of Marriages_1__ No. of Children_1__ Religion_Protestant____
Significant Historical Events:_Married 1940, son born 1949._
_____Traveled (camping) throughout U.S. with wife and son._
_____In Army, France WWII_____ Great bowler, won many trophies.__

INTERESTS
Please Specify: Past (P) or Current (C)
Art_____ Crafts_____ Cooking_____ Carpentry_woodworking_(P)
Games_cards P/C_ Music__P/C____ Instrument Played_guitar & mandolin_(P)
Animals__P/C__ Sports_P/C all__ Travel___P_____ Reading_newspapers_(P)
Volunteer Service or Social Clubs___Kiwanis (P)_____
Hobbies__bowling, woodworking, gardening (P)___ Gardening_raised veg._(P)
Other__bowling (P)_____
Socially Active?_always_Prefers Group or Individual Activity?_both__
____a very small circle of friends (P)_____Currently is quite isolated

COMMENTS

____Enjoys talking about his past, but currently has few interests. Spends

____most of the time alone in his apartment.

_____

_____

_____

Care Plan

Patient Care Plan

Patient's Name__Helen_____   Date__July 17_____
STAFF:_____Nursing:_____Soc. Wk:_____Activities:_____

PROBLEM	GOALS	PLAN & APPROACHES	STAFF
I. Physical			
Needs supervision in bathroom Unable to clean self	Keep her clean and free of odor & dry	Place her on bathroom list for supervision immediately and ongoing	R.N.
Possible limited mobility	Determine mobility status	Observe and record daily in progress notes by August 1	R.N. Actv.
II. Psychosocial			
Limited social contacts	Increase socialization by insuring at least one morning and one afternoon one-on-one	Special greeting upon arrival; introduce to other patients. Assign a volunteer, staff or patient to a minimum five minutes of conversation for morning and afternoon	Actv.
Limited ability to initiate activities or to be involved in activities	Will participate in planned center activities	Encourage with positive reinforcement when she participates and follows through in activities	Actv.
		Record participation on daily program sheet	Actv.
III. Family			
No contact with family	To develop regular contact with family	Set up an interview with family by August 1	SOC. WK.
		Invite family to group therapy sessions with psychiatrist	SOC. WK.

Monthly Review
Outcome:_____

Blank Care Plan

Patient Care Plan

Patient's Name_____   Date_____

STAFF:_____Nursing:_____Soc. Wk:_____Activities:_____

<u>PROBLEM</u>   <u>GOALS</u>   <u>PLAN & APPROACHES</u>   <u>STAFF</u>

I. <u>Physical</u>

II. <u>Psychosocial</u>

III. <u>Family</u>

Monthly Review
Outcome:_____

Basic Principles of

Positive Interaction

1. *In all interactions with patients, be pleasant, calm, and reassuring, to keep them feeling calm and reassured.* Dementia patients mirror the emotional climate around them. If others are upset, they will be upset. You must act the way you want them to act.

   a. Assess the patient. Try hard to understand how the patient must be feeling.

   b. Respond to these feelings. Show with your words, body language, and actions that you understand: validate the feelings as you also distract and reassure.

   • Get and maintain eye contact. Approach and stay in front of the person, where he or she can see what you are doing and saying.

   • Make sure your facial expression and body language are relaxed and pleasant and show your interest in the person.

   • Keep your tone of voice warm, pleasantly low, and fairly soft.

2. *Help patients maintain self-esteem.* Persons with dementia quite often realize that something is very wrong with them. They realize that they cannot perform and do not understand their environment as well as they did previously.

   a. Help the patient "save face." Avoid or simplify difficult activities, but always keep interactions on an adult level.

   b. If patients make errors or fail at a task, help them take it lightly. Assure them that no harm has been done. Avoid criticism.

c. Avoid negatives and commands.

d. Avoid "why" questions. Remember that they cannot reason well.

e. Give them the opportunity to make simple choices. This aids their sense of independence and self-esteem.

f. Set up a fairly structured routine. They then know what to expect. This aids short-term memory, increases their sense of independence, and reduces anxiety.

g. Help them use and enjoy their remaining strengths. Praise success.

3. *Always simplify the verbal message and accompany words with tactile and visual cues.*

a. Get and maintain eye contact; approach from the front and at eye level.

b. Use simple sentences consisting of only one idea or instruction.

c. Speak slowly.

d. Use gestures or props to help the patient understand.

e. Use touch to help the patient understand.

f. Repeat if needed. Do not go on to another idea or instruction until the persons grasps the first one.

Meaningful communication is a basic need of all human beings.

Understanding and Managing
the Catastrophic Reaction

1. Learn to identify a catastrophic reaction.

   Persons with dementia do not process and interpret environmental stimuli as well as the cognitively normal person. When they cannot understand the information they receive from their environment, or when they feel they are not understood, a catastrophic reaction can occur. It is a reaction of anger, fright, or frustration.

   They are *not* trying to annoy, get attention, or hurt the caregiver. They are *not* just lazy. They are trying their very best to deal with a world they cannot cope with anymore.

   A sudden behavior problem is the sign that a catastrophic reaction is taking place. A catastrophic reaction can be displayed through any of the following behaviors:

   verbal or physical aggression;

   verbal outbursts;

   worry;

   anger;

   tension in body language and
      facial expression;

   rapid change in mood;

   stubborn resistance;

   pacing or wandering;

   paranoia;

   crying;

   hysterical laughter;

   sudden self-isolation, refusal
      to speak.

2. If a catastrophic reaction occurs:

   a. Reassure.

b. Show the person you care: use open, friendly body language and tone of voice; speak respectfully and calmly. Don't let *your* anxiety show.

c. Be careful not to invade the person's "personal space" if he or she is extremely upset or angry.

d. Eliminate or reduce all outside stimulation.

e. Identify and remove the source of the problem or remove the person.

f. If the person is not extremely angry, or if he or she becomes calmer, a reassuring touch, a hug, or holding hands can be effective.

g. Redirect to a less-demanding, less-stressful activity. (Walk, talk reassuringly, look at pictures. This is not the time for a cognitively demanding activity such as a structured game, craft, etc.)

h. Be patient. Even if the person is responding to you, it often takes a while for him or her to calm down.

3. If you cannot minimize or stop the catastrophic reaction:

a. Leave the person alone if he or she is in a safe, quiet place. Being left alone may be what is needed. You may be adding to the distress without meaning to. If it is not safe for you to leave, back off so that the person can feel more alone, providing a "personal space."

b. If it has been necessary to leave a patient, when you come back, act as if nothing has happened. The short-term memory loss can work for you.

c. Use a "change of face." Have another person intervene. You should then leave. Two people gesturing and talking is confusing to a dementia patient, and you become part of the problem.

d. Try not to be upset or angry about anything a dementia patient says during a catastrophic reaction. Try not to feel as if you failed if another caregiver succeeds with a person and you cannot. Paranoia, inappropriate actions, verbal outbursts, and anger are symptoms of the dementia. Do not take them personally.

4. Afterward: Assess the cause of the catastrophic reaction. Perhaps the person was:

a. trying to comprehend more than one or two sensory messages at once, but could not;

b. feeling insecure;

c. having a minor mishap or failing at a task;

d. asked to reason or make a judgment (answer "why" questions, make complex choices);

e. experiencing negative interactions with others or had observed others scolding, arguing, or showing evidence of irritation, frustration, and anger;

f. misunderstanding or having delusions concerning the words and actions of people or events, or was hallucinating.

5. To avoid or minimize future catastrophic reactions:

   a. If the patient frequently has catastrophic reactions, review and assess the situations very carefully. Did the reactions usually occur at a certain time? Did the patient act a certain way just before the reactions occurred? If causes for the reactions can be identified and eliminated, perhaps they can be minimized or even avoided in the future.

   b. Always keep the environment calm. Avoid sensory overload.

   c. Simplify *all* tasks to ensure or increase the chance of success.

   d. Stick to a consistent routine, so that the person generally knows what to expect.

   e. Give the person plenty of time.

   f. Consistently use good interaction techniques.

HANDOUT II:2

Cue Card: The Management of Catastrophic Reactions

Put this quick reference on a 5″ × 7″ card and keep it in a handy place as a cue for interactions with dementia patients. Remember, *only* the main points are listed!

FRONT OF CARD:

Reminder!
The Management of Catastrophic Reactions

Sudden behavior change? Distract and reduce stimulation to keep a catastrophic reaction from happening!

If it occurs:

1. Reassure, using good interaction techniques. If the person is angry, reassure from a little distance!
2. Reduce all outside stimulation and hazards.
3. Identify and remove the problem or remove the person.
4. Reassure again. Use touch now if possible.
5. Redirect to a *less demanding* activity in a *quiet* place.
6. Be patient. It may take a while!

If you can't stop it:

1. Leave them alone if safe. Observe from a distance.
2. When they seem calmer, come back, act as if nothing happened, or use "change of face."
3. Afterward: Assess to avoid it in the future.

Remember: *Don't take it personally.* The reaction was a symptom of the disease.

Role-Playing Situations

Act out or discuss these situations. What would you do?

Role-Playing Situation 1: Avoiding a Catastrophic Reaction

THE ROLES

Class members 1 and 2: You are caregivers in a residential facility, responsible for care of residents with dementia.

Class member 3: You are a resident with a moderate degree of dementia. You refuse to dispose of a very soggy paper cup that held your soup at lunch. The leftover soup is dripping on the floor and is soiling your clothing. You continually insist that you need the cup and want to put it in your room. You are insistent but not catastrophic—at least, not yet.

Class member 4: You are a resident with a moderate degree of dementia sitting next to class member 3. You are telling class members 1 and 2 about the soggy cup. You are very upset about the soup dripping on the floor. You are telling them that resident 3 should be made to "Throw away that dirty cup!" You are moderately upset, but not catastrophic—at least, not yet.

THE TASK

Class members 1 and 2 are to resolve this problem with the two residents before they become even more anxious and upset.

Role-Playing Situation 2: Managing a Behavior Problem

THE ROLES

Class member 1: You are a nurse assistant in a skilled nursing facility unit for dementia patients. It is breakfast time and you come into the lounge area to let a new resident (class member 2) know that it is time for breakfast. The resident's chart states that he or she did not eat much the night before and did not socialize with other residents all day. You are concerned about his or her intake and adjustment to the facility.

Class member 2: You are a moderately impaired resident with dementia. You have been at the facility for only one week. You are adjusting slowly, but are still quite anxious and insecure at times. At breakfast time you do not wish to go into the dining room with the other residents. You are not angry, but you seem withdrawn.

THE TASK

Class member 1 is to try to get the new resident to eat at least some breakfast, hopefully with other residents.

Common Behavior Problems
of Persons with Dementia

Anxiety

Paranoia

Short attention span with minimal
ability to become reengaged

Outbursts: emotional, verbal, physically aggressive

Repetitive behaviors: actions, words,
or ideas

Hoarding

Suspiciousness

Rummaging

Wandering

Pacing

Depression

Day/night reversal

Nighttime activity

Apathy

Inappropriate sexual behavior

Other inappropriate social behaviors:
undressing in public, etc.

Hallucinations

Inappropriate toileting habits

Poor grooming habits: refusal
to bathe, brush hair, or brush
teeth

Refusal to eat

Eating too rapidly or too much

Eating nonfood items

Evaluating Problem Behaviors

for Effective Management

1. Is the behavior truly a problem?

    Is it harmful, potentially harmful, or upsetting to the person?
    Is it harmful, potentially harmful, or upsetting to others?
    Does it interfere with the person's ability or opportunity to perform alternate, more meaningful activities?

2. What is the problem?

    For best behavior management, problems must be carefully analyzed. There may be more than one problem. The primary problem must be identified. It may be the cause of others.
    Example: If a person wanders and rummages in closets and shelves, are both behaviors really problems? Does one cause the other?

3. When, where, and with whom does the problem behavior occur?

    Does it occur at a certain time of day?
    Does it occur in particular types of places or in certain types of situations (in overcrowded rooms, where there is lots of noise or activity)?
    Does a particular person (or persons) seem to trigger the problem more than others?

4. Why is the person behaving this way?

    Is the person uncomfortable physically? Is the person tired or ill? (Always assess the patient for physical problems first.)

Is the person having trouble communicating with the caregiver or others?

Is the person disoriented or misinterpreting the physical environment (hallucinations and delusions)?

Is the person in a new environment or situation?

Is the activity routine too unstructured? (Is there not enough to do or is there inadequate guidance?)

Is a task too demanding or unfamiliar?

The behavior may be a symptom of a certain stage of the dementia and may not have an external cause.

A person may not be able to stop a behavior before it becomes a problem: perseveration.

5. How can the behavior problem be managed?

Usually you cannot reason with the person with dementia. The person cannot voluntarily correct the behavior. The person will change the behavior only if he or she can be distracted to a more calming or pleasant alternative. With all other members of the caregiving team, decide on and try a specific course of action consistently for a while. (If it seems to be successful at all, try it for at least a day before giving up on the plan.) All caregivers involved must use the same techniques and communicate the results to each other.

Keep the patient physically comfortable.

Assess and change the daily schedule if needed: Does the person need more rest at night or rest periods during the day? Or, is the person too inactive? Are the current activities appropriate? Does the person need different, more meaningful, or less stressful activity?

Remove and keep away things in the environment (or other patients) that could be adding to or causing the problem. If the environment cannot be changed, provide alternate activities for the person in a different, controlled setting.

If the behavior seems to be occurring at a certain time of day, carefully choose activities and structure the environment to suit the person's needs at that time.

One member of the staff may have better luck with a person than another.

Be flexible. Try another plan if the first one doesn't work.

6. What do you do if you can't alleviate the problem?

Rotate staff members to distribute the burden of the person's care evenly among several caregivers.

Wait. The behavior may be a symptom of a certain stage of the disease and may change later.

Talk to the doctor. An unresolved medical problem may exist which might be causing the problem. Or, medication to alleviate the behavior problem may be possible. But, *try good behavior-management techniques first.*

Cue Card: Evaluating Recurring Behavior Problems

Put this quick reference on a 5″ × 7″ card and keep it in a handy place as a cue for interactions with dementia patients. Remember, *only* the main points are listed here!

Reminder!
The Evaluation of Recurring Behavior Problems

Assess as a team: Use the "who, what, when, where, why, and how" technique.

1. *Is* it really a problem?
2. *What* is the problem?
3. *When, where,* and *with whom* does it happen?
4. *Why* is it happening?
5. *How* can it be managed? As a team, decide on a very specific plan of action. All team members should use the technique consistently. Give it some time.
6. Reassess as a team. If the first technique didn't work, start again!

Case Studies: Behavior Problems

Dan (Hoarding)

Dan was a physically fit and healthy Alzheimer patient who attended an adult day care center on a daily basis. His neurological symptoms were generally Stage Two in severity. He was very social and loved to be with other people. He actively participated in all activities. He was amiable and when upset did not become visibly angry, but became stubborn and difficult to distract.

Dan had always become quickly absorbed in any activity going on and had trouble making a transition from one activity to another. For example, at Christmas one year, he became very absorbed in making paper Christmas chains (a good example of positive use of perseveration). He became visibly physically tired after about an hour but would not stop. The staff had to gently take the paper and glue from him and remove him from the table.

As the disease progressed, Dan's compulsive behavior became more extreme. He always brought a small leather satchel from home for personal belongings and also always wore a cap. He would put the cap in the bag when he wasn't wearing it. Several other men also wore caps and put them under their chairs or on a table when they were inside. Dan started taking the hats and would stuff them into his satchel. The behavior was a problem throughout the entire day and was a problem at home as well as at the center.

The problem quickly became worse. Dan would take any small item he saw lying around and put it in his satchel. When it was full, he stuffed his pockets. One day his pockets became so full, his trousers actually slipped to the floor.

What would you do to manage this situation? Before reading the management techniques we used, think of some of your own and then share ideas with your group, reaching a group decision. Use Handout II:6 as a guide to behavior evaluation and management.

The staff never *solved* the problem, but they did manage to keep it from upsetting Dan or the other patients severely. Techniques used included interventions by his wife and also by the staff:

1. Help from his wife:
   a. Dan's wife had him leave his satchel at home. She told him the satchel had been "lost." Dan became upset, but he enjoyed coming to the center, so he came without the satchel and soon forgot about it.
   b. Dan still put things in his pockets, so his wife sewed up the pockets.
   c. Dan then stuffed things inside his shirt and tucked them into his belt. She bought one-piece leisure suits *and* sewed up the pockets. This was quite effective, and though Dan would still grab things and hold onto them, he could not store them.

2. At the center:
   a. The staff thought of keeping Dan away from other patients. This really upset him, however. Staff members finally all just kept a close eye on him, moving things out of reach. They even occasionally asked him privately if they could check to see if he had put something "accidentally" in his pocket or jacket. The staff was afraid looking in his pockets would upset or embarrass him, but as it was done privately and it was stressed that items were "there by accident," he was never offended.
   b. The staff tried keeping a rummaging area just for Dan. This did not work, however. He would hoard all of those items and still go after other patients' belongings.
   c. The worst problem was with craft or art projects made by other patients. They liked to admire the projects after they were completed—a center art show. However, Dan would grab all the projects he could and stuff them in his satchel or jacket or just hold them. For a while, the staff decided to avoid displaying finished projects, but this was not fair to the other patients. Finally it was decided that projects would be displayed for a short time only, while one staff person took Dan on a walk away from the project area.

Diane and Edward (Inappropriate Sexual Behavior)

Diane and Edward are both healthy, very low Stage Two Alzheimer patients in their mid-sixties. They seem to have few remaining strengths and participate in hardly any of the activities at the residential care facility for the elderly where they live. Edward has some verbal skills remaining but refuses to be involved in any activities. Diane is aware of those around her but has extremely poor perceptual and organization-of-movement skills and very minimal receptive and expressive language ability.

HANDOUT II:8

They were attracted to each other as soon as they arrived at the facility. Smiles almost immediately escalated into public displays of sexual affection. They soon discovered where each other's rooms were and were found together frequently. Both are married, and their spouses visit very frequently. Diane and Edward exhibit this inappropriate behavior all day long but are not attracted to any of the other residents or staff.

What would you do to manage this situation? Before reading the management techniques actually used, think of some of your own and then share ideas with your group, reaching a group decision. Use Handout II:7 as a guide to behavior evaluation and management.

Sexual problems are difficult to manage. Spouses can be deeply hurt by a partner's inappropriate sexual attention to them or to others. They may be able to understand intellectually that the disease is causing the inappropriate behavior, but it may be very difficult for them to accept emotionally.

Dementia patients can suffer severe catastrophic reactions if they are in a sexual relationship that is not handled delicately and sensitively. A careless sexual encounter can cause panic, anger, or fear. They may not understand the feelings aroused and may not even understand what is happening.

As in the problem with Dan above, the staff never *solved* the problem, but they did manage to keep it from too severely upsetting Diane, Edward, their spouses, and the other residents. The problem with Diane and Edward was compounded by the fact that the staff originally did not want to tell either of the residents' spouses about it, since they did not want them to be hurt by the situation.

Management techniques used by the staff included:

1. Keeping Diane and Edward in separate groups for activities during the day. This was extremely difficult, however, because if they even briefly *saw* each other, they would want to be together. Luckily, the facility was large enough that they could be kept in different groups and even scheduled to eat at different times. In a very small facility, this would have been impossible.
2. Their rooms were placed at opposite ends of the facility. All night shift staff members were made aware of the problem and they made rounds of rooms more frequently.
3. Diane's husband was never informed of the problem, because the staff felt he was in such a precarious emotional state that he could not handle the situation well. Diane was quite young and was declining so very rapidly that her

husband was on the verge of an emotional breakdown. The staff referred him to counseling, and his therapist recommended that he visit her less frequently. This eased the situation for the staff as well.

4. Edward's wife had reached a greater level of acceptance of the disease process. She was told of the problem, accepted it, and actually helped. During her visits she made a point of helping the staff keep Diane and Edward apart, and Edward seemed aware of her presence and behaved more appropriately when she was there.

HANDOUT II:8

The problem eventually resolved itself when Diane reached such a level of severity that she was no longer attracted to Edward. He did not approach her once she no longer welcomed his attention.

Madeline (Repetitive Behaviors—Perseveration)

Refer to Handout I:9. Madeline's behavior problems and some techniques the staff tried in an attempt to manage these behaviors are listed there.

What would you do to manage these situations? Think of some management techniques of your own and share ideas with your group, reaching a group decision. Use Handout II:6 as a guide to behavior evaluation and management.

Medical Problems and the
Person with Dementia

1. General concerns

   People affected with dementia can also suffer from other chronic or acute diseases. Patients may not be able to tell you that they are in pain or to identify which part of their body hurts. Therefore, interpreting body language is vital.

   Example: A staff member noticed that Bill was limping during the daily walk. When he was asked if his leg was bothering him, the response was "No." Later that day Bill was sitting in a chair with his shoe off. A staff member took the opportunity to examine his foot and discovered an ulcer between the toes.

   When a person is observed to be more agitated or refuses to do an activity that is normally performed, he or she should be evaluated for possible injury or illness. Correcting a minor physical problem can often greatly reduce poor behavioral responses.

   Just as healthy people become mentally dull when ill, the person with dementia likewise experiences decreased abilities to cope and to successfully perform normal activities. Any indication of pain or illness should be taken seriously and not dismissed because the person suffers from dementia. Continuing consultation with a regular attending physician is just as vitally important with these patients as for a person with any other chronic progressive disease.

2. Symptoms of illness

   a. General symptoms requiring further evaluation:
      • Lips and gums that are pale, cyanotic, or dry
      • Refusal to eat or drink
      • Change in normal personality (e.g., irritability, drowsiness, withdrawal)
      • Change in behavior (e.g., refusal to do normal activities)
      • Disruptiveness
      • Headache, which may be observed as rubbing of the head or closing or squinting of the eyes
      • Twitching, convulsions, delirium, hallucinations, or unexplained falls
      • Swelling of any body part
      • Rapid respiration, coughing, or grunting, especially when trying to take a deep breath

   b. Fever. Aged persons usually have a lower-than-normal body temperature, so it's best to have a baseline for comparison. For example, an oral temperature of 99.8° F could be serious if the person's normal temperature is 97.6° F.

      When taking an oral temperature, be sure that the patient is not disoriented and is capable of keeping the thermometer in the mouth and under the tongue without biting it. Taking an axillary reading may be a better option. When taking an axillary reading, keep the thermometer in place for five minutes; the reading will be about 1 degree less than if it were being taken orally. The digital thermometer may be safer to use than the glass type.

   c. Abnormal skin. Observe for hot and dry, flushed or pale, cold or clammy skin. Dehydration may lead to a loss of skin elasticity. This can be checked by gently pinching the skin, preferably in the abdominal area in elderly persons. In a normal, well-hydrated person the skin will relax. If it remains rather pinched looking, poor hydration can be suspected.

      Elderly persons are prone to pressure sores because of decreased circulation and a tendency to be sitting or lying down for prolonged periods. They begin as reddened areas, usually over bony areas of the body. These areas can progress to deep oozing sores if not treated. Caregivers need to encourage the patient to change position frequently, and mild massages around the edges of the reddened areas may keep the condition from becoming serious.

   d. Vomiting and/or diarrhea. When these signs of illness occur, they may be indicative of minor stomach irritation, impacted stool, or more serious intestinal problems. Dehydration and electrolyte imbalance can develop very rapidly. The danger or aspiration is always present when vomiting occurs. Try to have the patient lie on his or her side or sit up and lean over when vomiting.

e. Irregular heartbeat. Increased, decreased, or irregular pulse rate is usually a significant sign that should be monitored and reported to the physician. A normal baseline with which to compare current readings is very helpful.

f. Constipation. A person should have a bowel movement at least every three days. A normal routine and consistency of the stool is more important than frequency. A dementia patient will probably not be able to tell you if he or she has had a bowel movement, and it is the caregiver's responsibility to monitor bathroom activities.

Constipation can lead to bowel impaction, and then a physician should be notified to determine treatment. Loose, liquid stools are a sign of impaction, along with excessive straining to pass a large fecal mass.

Constipation can be caused by a diet high in refined foods, poor fluid intake, less active bowel muscles, and certain medications. The following steps can be taken to prevent the problem, which will make things easier on the caregiver and the patient:

- Increase the intake of foods high in fiber
- Ensure adequate intake of fluids
- Ensure continuing exercise
- Administer stool softeners or bulking agents, mild laxatives, or enemas as ordered by the physician

Assisting the Dementia Patient
with Dressing

Many individuals afflicted with dementia like to layer clothing. Let them do this unless the weather is too hot or the family strongly disagrees.

Let the patient choose his or her clothes if possible; perhaps give an either/or selection. (Stretchy knits—leisure or jogging suits—are easy for caregiver and patient alike to remove.)

Avoid pantyhose; use socks, knee-highs, or thigh-highs instead. Stockings held up with circular garters may cut off the circulation to the lower leg.

Lay out clothes in the order they are to be put on, with underclothes on top and shoes on the bottom.

Supervise dressing but allow as much autonomy as possible.

Allow the patient plenty of time to dress. Don't rush him or her. This may lead to increased frustration, agitation, or combativeness.

If a problem arises, wait and/or approach the patient a little later.

Be patient. Allow plenty of time for simple tasks.

Due to damage in certain areas of the brain that control temperature regulation, the dementia patient may feel cold when the temperature seems warm to others. Allow the patient to dress for comfort (within reason). Observe for perspiration.

Some individuals may be taking medication that causes increased sensitivity to the sun; check patients' medical records before taking them outside. They may need to wear a hat or use a sun-blocking lotion.

Make sure that the patient's shoes are tied securely.

If the patient is incontinent, encourage the use of pants with elastic waistbands, which are easier to change.

Nutritional Concerns for Persons with Dementia

Problems with eating, drinking, chewing, and swallowing associated with Alzheimer disease and similar dementing disorders can make mealtime very difficult for the patient and very trying for you. Yet, as many caregivers have learned from experience, if patients sense your exasperation or feel hurried or pressured, their agitation and eating problems are likely to increase. To avoid major problems, try to adhere to a constant mealtime routine, serving at regular hours each day and in the customary way each mealtime. Maintain as calm and pleasant an atmosphere as possible.

Inability to chew is a frequent source of difficulty for elderly persons because of poorly fitting dentures or an absence of teeth. With decreased ability to chew, you may have to serve soft or pureed foods such as applesauce, bananas, scrambled eggs, mashed potatoes, ground meat, or cottage cheese. People with dementing illnesses may forget how to chew. Do not give them foods they may forget to chew thoroughly, such as nuts, popcorn, pretzels, small hard candies, carrots, grapes, or cherries with pits.

Sometimes people with coordination problems begin to have trouble swallowing. If the person has difficulty changing facial expression, he or she may also have trouble chewing or swallowing. When this occurs, it is important to guard against choking. Soft, thick foods are less likely to cause choking. Avoid the combination of liquids and solids, such as ready-to-eat cereals and cold milk. This may cause choking. The two textures, liquid and solid, make it difficult for the person to know whether to chew or swallow. Make note of whether solids or liquids cause problems; often liquids cause problems because they are swallowed too quickly.

If the patient has forgotten how to feed himself or herself or is having trouble coordinating his or her actions, try "patterning": take the spoon and place food on it; then put the spoon in the patient's hand. Gently help the patient to guide the spoon into his or her mouth. Remind the person to chew and swallow. Repeat this process and at the same time praise the person's ability to feed himself or herself independently. This technique can be useful with other behavior problems as well as with eating. If this doesn't work, serve finger foods (sandwiches cut into small pieces; raw fruits and vegetables cut into slices), which are easier to handle. If necessary, remind the person to swallow each bite. Offer fluids after every three to four mouthfuls of solid foods, to help wash the food down.

Appetite usually declines in later years. The ultimate cause is yet unknown, but it may be because the senses of smell and taste and are less acute. Serve four or five small meals when appetite is poor. Foods should be well flavored, not bland—but not too highly seasoned with very strong spices, since older stomachs can be upset more easily.

Memory-impaired persons appear to lose their sense of hot and cold and may burn their mouths on hot foods and drinks. Always test the temperature of foods and drinks before serving. Don't insist that a person eat or drink if he or she is sleepy or irritable. Return the food to the kitchen and try again later. Missing one meal is not a calamity; insisting that a person eat may cause one. Don't allow the person to walk around or to lie down with food in his or her mouth. Conversation makes a meal more pleasant, but avoid too much—it can be distracting.

Many choices of food on a plate confuse an impaired person. Serve one part of the meal at a time. Keep the number of forks, spoons, and knives to a minimum. Sometimes a spoon is sufficient, and the lack of choice discourages playing with the silverware.

An impaired person may have forgotten the concept of "food" and may eat things that look like food. Dog biscuits, artificial flowers or fruit, or anything colorful that resembles food may become the meal of the day.

Elderly people sometimes experience reduced production of saliva. Medications often cause drying of the mouth. To compensate for this deficiency, serve moist food and liquids with each meal. Be sure the person drinks fluids each day, especially during warm weather.

Use a bendable straw. Many individuals who won't or can't drink are still able to suck through a straw.

Due to loss of coordination, a person with dementia can become a messy eater. He or she may spill food and beverages frequently. To decrease the amount of clean-up, use a plastic tablecloth and have the person wear an attractive plastic or waterproof apron. You may also want to serve the food in a bowl instead of on a plate. This may make it easier for the person to maneuver the food onto the spoon.

A patient may want to eat all the time, even if he or she has just finished a meal. Try reducing the portions you serve at meals and provide in-between meal snacks of fruit or yogurt.

If the patient must be fed, offer small bites and remind him or her to chew and swallow as needed. If the patient bites down on the utensil, don't use plastic and don't try to remove it forcibly. Ask the person to open his or her mouth or wait until the muscles of the jaw tire and relax.

Oral Care

Oral care for dementia patients can be very frustrating. It is difficult for the care provider to show patients what needs to be done inside the mouth, and patients have difficulty comprehending verbal instructions that may be fairly complex. In addition, psychotropic medications often prescribed for behavior management can alter salivary function and lead to diminished oral health.

Even higher-functioning dementia patients may have trouble identifying the location of mouth pain and will probably be unable to identify areas of the mouth which feel inadequately cleaned or have food particles adhering. The care provider must regularly assess each individual patient's mouth condition. In addition, the need for assistance should be evaluated, remembering that some patients retain long-term memory and habitual skills better than others. Each patient will require different types of cues and a different degree of assistance. The care provider must develop an individualized program of care before proceeding.

Oral care *twice daily* is part of the daily care of *every patient.* This includes care of the mouth, teeth, gums, and tongue. Not only health but also self-esteem is involved, since soiled teeth and gums and foul odor can repulse others. Day care providers, even though they are not the primary care providers, should feel obligated to assist families as needed with oral care. More frequent visits to the dentist to *prevent* problems may be easier than caring for major dental problems later.

A mouth in poor condition can be a cause of decreased appetite and fluid intake. While performing dental care, watch for and report:

1. sores in the mouth;
2. loose or broken teeth;
3. bleeding;
4. bad mouth odor.

Steps to follow for proper oral care:

1. Assess the person's mouth condition daily and reevaluate the person's ability to perform self-care regularly. Let patients perform as much of the task themselves as possible, as long as they can do a thorough job.
2. Wear gloves.
3. Make sure the person is comfortable.
4. Use a soft, junior-size brush. This permits thorough cleaning without gum damage. Encourage independent brushing. A special easy-grip handle or one wrapped with foam may help.
5. Approach the person using good positive interaction techniques. Show the person what you need to do as simply as possibly, *one step at a time.* Use visual (showing the implements, perhaps pointing in your own mouth and showing them in the mirror) and tactile cues.
6. Make sure the person understands one step to the best of his or her ability before you proceed to the next step. Don't rush the person. This can increase confusion and agitation.
7. If dentures are used, help the person to remove them first. (Remember to let the patient know what you are doing!) Clean appropriately.
8. Use a dry brush to help stimulate gums *very gently* first. Use a circular motion.
    a. Massage where the teeth and gums meet.
    b. Brush upper teeth first (brushing lower teeth causes excess saliva).
    c. Brush outer, inner, and chewing surfaces.
9. After about one and a half minutes, repeat this process using toothpaste.
10. Report any bleeding when rinsing.
11. Avoid the use of fluoride rinses, because patients may swallow them. Fluoride gels may work effectively.
12. *Always* remove dentures at night.

The Use of Dentures and

Other Assistive Devices

The use of dentures and other assistive devices (such as hearing aids and glasses) is often difficult with dementia patients. It is somewhat easier if the patient has used the device for a long time, but difficulty increases when the patient uses the device for the first time after the onset of dementia.

The use of *any* device that can increase sensory input and help the person function more easily should be encouraged. However, as dementia becomes very severe, the patient may become agitated or obsessed with the device. The caregiver must then evaluate the benefit of continued use versus discontinuation.

Patients cannot evaluate the comfort, proper fit, and effectiveness of assistive devices for themselves. The care provider and professional who prescribed the device must evaluate it frequently.

If the patient uses dentures, the care provider must be alert to changes in eating habits, behavior, weight, and health, since these symptoms may be signs of poorly fitting dentures.

If the patient uses a hearing aid or glasses, the caregiver must watch for decreased perceptual abilities and attention span. These symptoms could be caused by changes in vision or hearing rather than by increased severity of the dementia.

The care provider should monitor any assistive device several times daily to see if it is inserted and/or worn properly, functioning correctly, and not causing any tissue damage.

Incontinence

The incontinent patient may be aware of feelings of embarrassment and humiliation. He or she may feel frustrated and angered by the need to depend on others for the most basic needs.

Incontinence for an adult can result in loss of self-esteem. When the patient is incontinent, it is best to treat the situation in a matter-of-fact manner and always with understanding and empathy. Scolding or judging the person will only increase his or her discomfort. After each accident it is important to wash and dry the person's skin thoroughly, to prevent irritation and sores.

Urinary incontinence can be due to a number of causes:

1. The person may forget how to respond to signals from the bladder that tell him or her it needs emptying.
2. The person may be unable to get to the bathroom quickly enough.
3. The person may forget what the bathroom is for.
4. A person who urinates in wastepaper baskets, drawers, closets, or other inappropriate places may be unable to find the bathroom.

Establishing a regular routine can decrease and perhaps eliminate incontinence. Take the patient to the bathroom every two or three hours. You may find from observing the person that certain clues in behavior or speech let you know that he or she needs to urinate. (For example, a man may be tugging at his pants or opening his fly.) Anytime the person is restless or wandering about and seems to be looking for something, ask the person if he or she needs to use the bathroom. The person may have a special word for the bathroom/toilet; ask the family or caregiver to help you understand him or her.

If the patient wears a protective garment, be sure you check it routinely. A garment saturated with urine or feces can irritate the skin and lead to urine burns and open sores. Dispose of soiled protective garments in a plastic bag. Secure the bag so that there is no odor. If a urinal is used, be sure to rinse it out with water.

Always wash your hands thoroughly after assisting the patient.

The Management of Sleep Disturbances
Common among Persons with Dementia

At one time or another, most people with a dementing illness will experience sleep disturbances. The following points may help caregivers understand and cope with this problem.

1. The adult's need for sleep decreases with age: less REM sleep is needed and more wakefulness occurs. In the person with dementia, the normal aging changes are exaggerated, and nighttime wandering frequently occurs.
2. Try to decrease activity a few hours before bedtime, to prevent overstimulation. A quiet time listening to music or watching television calms the person.
3. Try to avoid nighttime fluids and diuretics, to prevent the person from needing to use the toilet during the night. (Coffee, tea, and cola act as diuretics.)
4. Try to lessen the fear and disorientation that may occur when the person awakens by using a night light in the bedroom.
5. Keep the person with dementia from napping during the day. Engage him or her in a regular daily exercise routine to relieve stress and boredom.
6. Avoid foods high in sugar after dinner: they tend to act as a stimulant. Try offering a glass of warm milk instead.
7. Orient and direct the patient back to bed using good positive interaction techniques. A confrontation will only aggravate the problem.
8. Examine your facility for safety hazards if night wandering occurs. Secure all windows (licensed care facilities need to consult with their department of

licensing on this) and use door alarms. A staff member should be alert and watchful for wanderers at all times.

9. If all else fails and sleep disturbances continue, explain the problems clearly to the physician and discuss the possibility of sleep medication.

BY SUSAN REED-WADE, R.N., ESCONDIDO GEORGE G. GLENNER ALZHEIMER'S FAMILY CENTER.

HANDOUT II:15

Assisting the Dementia Patient with Bathing

The caregiver must assess the patient's ability to bathe independently and should allow the patient to do as much as possible.

If the patient is independent and just needs simple direction, the caregiver should arrange bathing items in the order in which they are to be used. Items for each task should be set out as they are needed. For example, soap, washcloth, and towel for a shower should be set out first. Items for shaving should be set out only after the shower is completed. The caregiver must remember always to use good interaction techniques. Directions should be simple and repeated as necessary.

The water temperature of a tub bath or shower should always be checked, and the pressure of a shower should be gentle. A hand-held shower rather than an overhead shower is usually less frightening. (Decreased circulation and cognitive functioning may inhibit a patient's ability to judge water temperature and to deal with a hard flow of water directly overhead.)

Tub bathing should be attempted only if the individual is agile enough to get in and out of the tub independently. The water should be no deeper than five inches. In most cases, the caregiver should stay with the patient throughout the bath. Rubber mats should be used to prevent slipping. Bath oils should be used with care or avoided, as they can make the floor slippery.

The caregiver should use the bath time to assess the person's skin for any infections, rashes, or swellings. Because of the dementia, the patient may not be able to tell the caregiver of any problems. The caregiver should always check the genital area and make sure it is washed thoroughly to prevent odors and skin breakdown.

When cleaning the patient's ears, the caregiver should avoid sticking any objects into the ear. The finger-and-washcloth method should be used. The caregiver should check the outer ear canal for excessive drainage, which can indicate acute ear infection or hearing problems.

The patient should be encouraged to dress attractively after bathing. A person feels good after a bath; even the simple act of putting on a clean and attractive robe before going to bed increases morale and self-esteem.

When helping the patient to brush his or her teeth, the caregiver should try to keep to a routine that feels familiar to the patient. (See "Oral Care," Handout II:12.) Step-by-step directions must be used. The caregiver should try to get the person to clean his or her mouth after each meal with baking soda, toothpaste, or at least fresh water.

BY SUSAN REED-WADE, R.N., ESCONDIDO GEORGE G. GLENNER ALZHEIMER'S FAMILY CENTER.

The Role of Psychotropic Medications in Modifying Inappropriate Behaviors of Dementia Patients

The use of psychotropic medications for modifying behaviors can be a two-edged sword. Medications can play a vital role in helping the dementia patient to sleep or to control agitation, but at the same time the person is vulnerable to overmedication as well as to adverse reactions from combinations of drugs. No current medication will stop the degenerative process of Alzheimer disease or produce permanent improvement in functioning level. However, medication can often control some symptoms and improve the patient's quality of life and—temporarily, at least—functioning level. This should always be the goal for the use of psychoactive medication.

Medications currently available for behavior modification may also, however, have side effects, which Alzheimer patients may be unable to report. This means that caregivers should watch for these potential problems.

Side effects that caregivers should check for include:

drowsiness, lethargy;
increased confusion;
problems with ambulation, vertigo, ataxia;
incontinence;

hallucinations;
agitation;
constipation;
rash;
hypotension.

Also try to assess accurately whether the medication has truly helped with the management of the behavior problems being observed. Is the patient really more manageable, less anxious, more alert, etc.? Do the negative side effects of the medication outweigh the benefits?

When administering medications, avoid complex explanations of why the medication is needed. Simply state that it may "make you feel better" or that "it will keep you from feeling ill." Again, positive interaction techniques are vital. Use simple, one-step directions and maintain a warm, positive, matter-of-fact attitude.

HANDOUT II:17

If you don't succeed in giving the medication, try again later or have someone else approach the patient. Never try to force medication on someone.

Be sure to check that the patient has swallowed the pill. If the person is unable to swallow pills, check to see if the medication comes in a liquid form. You may need to crush the pill and add it to food.

Remember always to try nonpharmacological treatment of behavior difficulties before requesting medication for them. Medication should be given on a regular basis to achieve a reliable, constant low level of the drug in the body. Medication should not be given only when agitation occurs. It takes time for a medication's effectiveness to build up. Larger doses will be required if it is given sporadically.

PORTIONS BY SUSAN REED-WADE, R.N., ESCONDIDO GEORGE G. GLENNER ALZHEIMER'S FAMILY CENTER.

Drugs in the Management of Persons with Dementia: An Overview

Medications can play an important role in the care of patients with Alzheimer disease. Tacrine (Cognex) has been shown to produce modest, *transient* improvement in memory in some (perhaps 20 percent of) patients with mild to moderate Alzheimer disease. (It has not been studied in other dementias, and no effect is to be expected.) Because it is quite toxic (pharmacological effects include nausea, diarrhea, incontinence, and seizures; and there is chemical toxicity to the liver in roughly 30 percent of patients), not all Alzheimer patients will tolerate it. There is no evidence to suggest that it slows the degenerative process in the brain. In controlled studies, generally slightly fewer than half of the patients are able to tolerate the drug in dosages that might be effective.

While no current medication will stop the degenerative process or produce clinically important improvement in the thinking and memory of most dementia patients, drug treatment may calm agitation and help relieve some of the confusion caused by dementia. The benefits may include reduced anxiety, more restful sleep, and increased ability to enjoy activities. Another important benefit of medication may be to allow an agitated patient to become accustomed to a new environment, such as an Alzheimer family center or a special dementia care unit. Once familiar with the new surroundings, the patient can benefit from the stimulation and socialization the program provides (and often the medication can be discontinued).

Despite their often dramatic benefits, the medications currently available for behavior problems of persons with dementia often have limiting side effects.

Because Alzheimer patients may have difficulty describing their symptoms, often it will not be clear whether an observed behavior problem is due to a drug, or to an unrelated medical problem (such as a urinary tract infection or pain from arthritis), or is simply part of the variable course of the disease. Thus, careful observation by knowledgeable professionals and concerned family members is crucial to the successful use of medication for dementia.

The basic principles of drug therapy are as follows:

1. Obtain an accurate diagnosis.
2. Establish treatment goals.
3. Try nondrug treatments first.
4. Pick the most appropriate drug for the problem.
5. Tailor the chosen drug to the individual (with attention to other medical problems, such as heart disease, Parkinson disease, orthostatic hypotension, sleep disturbance, and other medications).
6. In most outpatient settings, start with low doses.
7. Keep it simple.
8. Educate the patient and caregivers on how to administer the drug and what effects and side effects to expect.
9. Evaluate the treatment for effects, both beneficial and adverse. (Systematic observation is critical.)
10. Change the therapy if indicated. Can any drug be stopped?
11. Keep drugs in a locked cabinet so that dementia patients cannot take them accidentally.

These steps require careful observation by caregivers and close coordination and evaluation by the primary treating physician. Experienced medical supervision is crucial. Consult the doctor about drug prescribing and treatment changes.

For example, Mrs. Thompson begins attending an Alzheimer family center. Despite a few days of one-to-one staffing to help her get oriented, she still becomes very agitated in the new environment and is unable to participate in center activities. The treatment goal for Mrs. Thompson is to calm her agitation and confusion so that she can become familiar with and feel comfortable in the center and enjoy its activities. Since nonpharmacological treatment (intensive staff support) has failed with Mrs. Thompson, the use of medications to reduce her agitation and the disordered thoughts that accompany it is indicated.

Administering the medicine on a regular basis each morning (or evening) can achieve a reliable, constant, but low, level of the drug in the body. This is more likely to provide sustained control of confusion than usage "as needed." It will be more effective than waiting until agitation becomes a major problem before giving the drug. If the caregiver waits until agitation is well under way, larger doses of the drug are needed, the patient and caregivers are more stressed by waiting for the drug to work, and, because larger doses are used, side effects are more likely.

Generally, I would prescribe a *low dose* of an antipsychotic agent or trazodone in this situation, when behavioral interventions have failed. The antipsychotic agents are favored when there are delusions (fixed false beliefs), paranoia, or hallucinations, though in low doses they may be helpful for confusion. If the patient already has some Parkinsonian features (such as shuffling gait, difficulty turning or getting up from a chair, stiffness, etc.), I try to avoid prescribing antipsychotic drugs (unless required for psychotic symptoms). In general, benzodiazepines (such as diazepam [Valium], lorazepam [Ativan], etc.) tend to disinhibit dementia patients and may lead to increased confusion and behavior problems.

Antipsychotic and antidepressant medications build up slowly in the body. After several days to a week of treatment, the effects must be evaluated. If intolerable side effects have occurred, the medication should be stopped. In such a case, a drug with a different spectrum of side effects can be tried. If the medication has not resulted in calmer behavior, then the dosage needs to be slowly and systematically increased. Consistent, systematic changes in the dosage, allowing time for the full accumulation of the drug to occur, accompanied by systematic observation of behavior is crucial to effective drug treatment for persons with dementia. Due to fluctuations in the dementia itself, varying environmental irritations, and the slow elimination of most drugs used for these problems, daily changes in the dosage are unwarranted and are unlikely to lead to a stable, effective treatment regimen.

ADAPTED WITH PERMISSION FROM J. EDWARD JACKSON, M.D., ASSOCIATE PROFESSOR OF MEDICINE AND ASSOCIATE CLINICAL PROFESSOR OF PHARMACOLOGY, DIRECTOR, SENIORS ONLY CARE CLINIC, UNIVERSITY OF CALIFORNIA, SAN DIEGO.

Common Sensory Problems of Aging and Environmental Modifications to Assist and Support

Common Problems	Environmental Modifications
VISION PROBLEMS	
Objects are not seen as clearly, difficulty adjusting to near and far vision changes and to changes in lighting levels	Use large print Use contrasting colors Make sure rooms are well lit Use dimmer switches and three-way bulbs to adjust lighting levels Try to maintain steady lighting levels without shadows
Cannot see as well in low levels of illumination	Use outdoor light Increase lighting levels Mix fluorescent and incandescent lighting Use bulbs that provide natural lighting
Difficulty judging distance	Use color contrast on stairs Avoid sudden changes in levels (room entries down one step) Avoid strong color contrasts on floors, which can look like changes in level

Common Problems	Environmental Modifications
Increased sensitivity to glare	Adjust or change shades on bulbs that glare Use blinds, sheers, or drapes on windows Reduce floor shine

HEARING PROBLEMS

Reduced ability to hear high-frequency sounds and to distinguish between types of sounds (live and recorded voices or background noise and voices)	Reduce the bass on sound equipment In conversation areas, reduce background noise such as TV, recorded recorded announcements, telephone, dishwasher Use acoustical materials on surfaces

TACTILE DECLINE

Touch does not decrease as early as hearing and vision, but eventually does decline	Provide lots of different textures indoors and out Thicker or larger pages in books, easy-grip handles, larger buttons and buttonholes or other types of closures may be useful

DECLINE IN SENSES OF TASTE AND SMELL

Taste and smell, like touch, do not decline as rapidly as vision and hearing, but do decline eventually	Use herbs and spices to maximize the sense of taste. Make table colorful, pleasant to encourage appetite Avoid very hot or extremely cold foods to avoid mouth injury Encourage recognition and appreciation of food smells and fragrances. Use fragrant flowers and herbs in the garden

COMMON PROBLEMS WITH MOBILITY, POSTURE, AND LARGE- AND FINE-MOTOR STRENGTH

Stooped posture, slowness, stiffness in joints, limited movement of limbs	Use lever handles and easy-grip implements Avoid sudden changes in level

Use grab bars and rails for support wherever needed

Use nonskid mats in bathrooms and in slippery outdoor areas

Avoid low furniture, sharp corners

Design open, wide paths indoors and out

Place items used regularly on lower, easy-to-reach shelves

For easier gardening, use raised garden beds

Provide easy-on and -off clothing

Note: Overall physical changes common to aging and some causes of the changes are discussed in Module I.

Environmental Changes to Consider in Your Care Setting

No care setting is perfect, no matter how well it is designed. There is always a way to make things work better. Think about all areas of your care facility independently. Consider:

each living area;	stairs and ramps;
bedrooms, if applicable;	entrance areas;
bathrooms;	yard and outdoor walkways.
hallways;	

Are there things that could be dangerous, confusing, upsetting, or uncomfortable for dementia patients in any of these areas? Consider the following questions for each area. If any of your answers would be "No," what changes could you make for the better?

1. Is the area pleasing and homelike? Does it provide positive stimulation for the senses?
2. Does the area provide adequate environmental cues to assist dementia patients in:
   • orientation?
   • wayfinding?
   • using the environment appropriately?
3. Is the area as safe as possible? Is it adapted for easy surveillance?

Some environmental changes are not expensive to make. If it does seem that major, expensive changes are needed, brainstorm with other care providers. Perhaps less-expensive solutions are possible. If problems have to do with safety, they *must be taken care of immediately.* If they do not, perhaps expensive changes can be made in stages as money becomes available.

"Top Priorities" List

List things that need to be changed in your care setting:	List how you would go about making the change:
1.	
2.	
3.	

Comfortable Seating Is Essential

The person in the drawing on the left below can easily rise independently from the chair without assistance. The chair is just the right depth. The point at which her knees bend is just past the chair's front edge, so the thighs have good support but the knees can still bend appropriately. The feet comfortably touch the floor, indicating that the chair is the right height. The arms of the chair extend for its full depth and are of a good height to provide proper leverage when she rises.

The unfortunate person in the drawing on the right will probably not be able to rise without help. If he eventually does, it will take a lot of scooting and wiggling, and he may understandably be very irritable when he finally gets up! The chair is too deep. His knees cannot bend and awkwardly stick out in front of

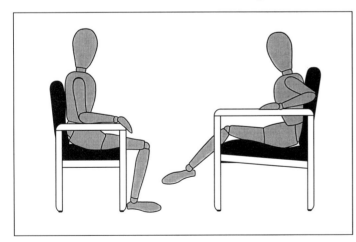

him. The chair is also slightly too high. The armrests are almost at shoulder height and do not provide any leverage for getting up. They would also impede his freedom of movement while in the chair.

Remember that chairs should be soft enough to be comfortable but not too soft to impede movement in them. Armrests are needed for stability in sitting and rising, but they should allow freedom of movement and should be padded for comfort. Chairs should be straight for work at a table or for exercise.

Floor Plan Guide: Dementia Care Unit
or Small, Freestanding Residential Facility

The small "home" on the next page can be a separate wing of a larger facility; one of several small wings in a facility, perhaps connected to a large lobby area by hallways (like spokes around the center of a wheel); or a small, freestanding residential facility. It could be for twelve residents in double rooms or for six residents in single rooms.

1. Entrance: This is the main entrance to the home. It is into the office, to avoid disturbing residents' daily routines and to control visitors.

2. The office: The office is small. Staff members are encouraged to stay with patients, *not* to observe from the office. It should have a *complete view* of the large patient activity area, kitchen, and quiet area through glass or over half-partitions. If glass is used, decals or division of large glass areas into smaller panes is necessary to avoid injuries. If partitions are used, shutters could be used above the partitions to shut off the area completely for private meetings.

3. The kitchen: Food preparation and the sounds and smells of cooking are familiar and pleasing to patients. To shut off the kitchen while allowing for visibility and interaction between staff in the kitchen and patients, half-doors, half-dividers, and shutters could be used. (In a larger facility, this area might be used for cooking activities and snack preparation only; resident meals would be prepared by the dietary department in another location.) *Note:* Avoid large windows in all rooms at the front of the building (2–4), since this area looks out onto the building's entrance area and could trigger anxiety and wandering by residents. High windows and skylights could be used instead.

4. The quiet room: This small area next to the kitchen is intended for very small groups, as a quiet room for agitated residents, or for family visits. Half-partitions and shutters could be used for controlled access and visibility from the main activity area. The preparation of snacks and some simple meal items is an activity that most patients enjoy. Therefore, when food preparation is intended as a large-group patient activity, it should be done in the large central activity area.

5. Storage rooms: These three wedge-shaped areas can be used as storage accessed from the quiet room and/or from the outside.

6. Residents' rooms: Note that all residents' rooms have clear views of the large activity area and of the outside yard, to encourage active participation by residents. This helps avoid the "out of sight, out of mind" problem.

7. The main activity area: This large area is clearly visible from the two staff duty areas—the office and the kitchen—as well as from residents' rooms. It can be used as one large room for large groups and large-motor activities or broken up into smaller areas (important at mealtime). Sound-reduction measures should be taken in walls, floor, and ceiling. Activity cabinets and a sink should be placed along some walls where they are easily accessible.

8. These four "wedges" are six-foot acoustically treated dividers on wheels (which should be locked once they are positioned). They can be placed as illustrated for meals or small, quiet activities, when reduced visual and auditory stimulation are needed. The staff in the kitchen and office retain some view of the room even when the dividers are up, because there are spaces between them. The dividers can be used in any way desired to break up the large activity area into smaller spaces. When not in use, they can be folded against side walls (walls can contain recessed areas so that the dividers can be slid into them and stored evenly with the rest of the wall).

9. The activity room path: A path for active wanderers and those just out for a stroll is necessary. This circular walkway allows residents a safe, unobstructed path within the facility.

10. The patio: The patio, path, and yard beyond are fully visible from the staff office and kitchen, the main activity area, and patients' rooms when dividers are not in use. The outside wall should be made of well-marked glass panes for view of the yard area.

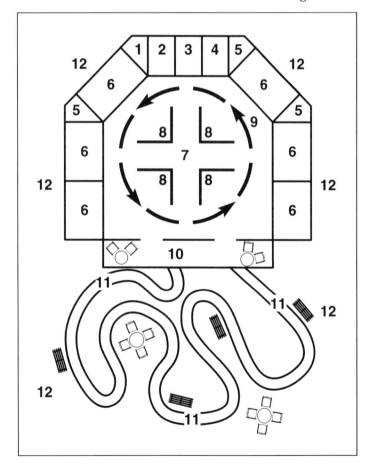

The patio should be covered to control glare, heat, and skin damage by the sun.

11. The outdoor paths: The wide, level paths avoid any sharp angles and leave from and return directly to the patio. The frame of the patio door could also be painted a bright contrasting color so that it is clearly visible to anxious walkers. Note that seating is included strategically along the path, to encourage rest and a break from a wandering pattern. Flower and vegetable beds should also be planted (remember to have raised beds).

12. The yard area: The grassy yard should be tree shaded and completely enclosed by at least a ten-foot fence, which should also screen views of the surrounding area (a locked gate for emergency exits might be necessary at the bottom of the property). Since residents' rooms look out onto side yards, these areas should also be attractive and effectively fenced and screened.

The Design and Positioning of Furniture

The design and positioning of furniture in an area should be appropriate to its use. The large room diagramed below is organized into four activity areas. The zigzag lines indicate movable dividers, which reduce auditory and visual confusion. Chairs in all areas are angled for best advantage in the activity to be presented there.

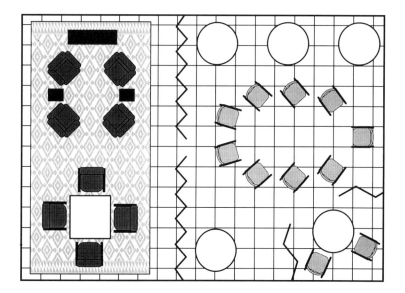

The left side of the room is defined by a rug (well anchored and not too soft, since toes can catch). It is set up for quiet conversation and reading. Each pair of armchairs has a table between them for coffee, the newspaper, etc.

The small table below the conversation area is set up for a game of cards or other tabletop activity. Chairs are sturdy straight backs with arms.

The large open area on the other side of the divider is set up for a large group activity such as exercise, or for a discussion group or some sort of large-group word game. Flooring is cushioned tile, which makes for more comfortable footing and reduced noise levels. If set up for exercise, note that chairs are far enough apart to allow for large arm movement and standing exercises, as appropriate. All chairs are angled toward the group leader. Tables for eating, crafts, etc., have been pushed to the side of the room *out of the way* of the activity group.

The small table in the lower right corner is in a quiet area with a small divider. Note that the two chairs are angled toward the large activity group for a solitary patient and a staff person. They are positioned with a view of the group, since the patient may decide to participate after all if given a few minutes alone to calm down or get used to the idea.

Magical Transformations:

Now You See It, Now You Don't!

Now you see it! A feeling of belonging is very important for dementia patients. They become anxious and worried when they can't find their way around. If they cannot find their room—their own special place—anxiety can be very severe. The door on the right below gives very important clues to a patient that it is his or her room. The door is highlighted. The border stripe on the floor ends on either side of the door. The room number is very large and at an appropriate height for easy visibility. The patient's name is in very large print on the door and a photo that is *meaningful to him or her* is also attached. Next to the door is a display box of items which the patient is proud of as well. It not only

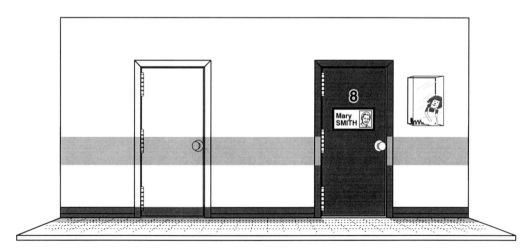

orients the patient to the room but can also be a topic of conversation with those passing by.

Now you don't! There are many rooms in a care setting to which patient access should be limited. These include storage areas, bathing rooms, offices, and the kitchen, among others. Patients do not usually understand *why* they cannot enter an area, however, so camouflage is often the most effective means of control. It uses the "out of sight, out of mind" principle. In the left of the drawing, the decorative stripe on the wall is continued over the door *and* the handle is painted to match. The border stripe on the hallway floor continues directly in front of the door as a visual barrier to entry. If some sort of signage is needed, it should be small and very inconspicuous.

HANDOUT III:6

Sources for Adaptive Equipment

Local hardware stores and medical supply stores may have good ideas for you and many of the supplies you need to purchase.

Some catalogs include:

1. *Adaptability: Products for Independent Living*, P.O. Box 515, Colchester, CT 06415-0515. Tel. 800 243-9232.

2. *Enrichments: Catalog for Easier Living*, P.O. Box 5050, Bolingbrook, IL 60440. Tel. 800 343-9742.

3. *HIP: Help for Incontinent People*, P.O. Box 544, Union, SC 29379. Tel. 800 BLADDER. (HIP publishes a helpful newsletter, which also advertises products. It costs $10.00.)

4. *ADL: Products for the Activities of Daily Living*, North Coast Medical, Inc., 187 Stauffer Boulevard, San Jose, CA 95125-1042. Tel. 800 821-9319.

5. *Mountainville House Calls*, P.O. Box 331148, Fort Worth, Texas 76163-1148. Tel. 800 460-7282.

Surveillance Systems to Assist with Monitoring Ambulatory Dementia Patients

Patients with Alzheimer disease and related types of dementia are frequently quite healthy physically and need to remain active. To reduce the necessity for active intervention by caregivers, large open areas free from safety hazards and a variety of safe yet satisfying activities must be provided. Patients need to continue to walk about freely and engage in meaningful activity.

Surveillance devices can make the restriction and monitoring of patients as they move about less invasive for patients and easier for care providers. They alert a care provider if the patient leaves a secure area. These alarm systems range very simple types to complex, extremely sensitive models. Prices range from $8.00 to thousands of dollars. Rentals and leases are also available. A few of the many systems available are:

1. *Care-Trak*, 1031 Autumn Ridge Road, Carbondale, IL 62901. Tel. 618 549-6330. They have a device that constantly monitors a building and outside area, emitting a signal when a person being monitored is missing. Patients can wear the transmitter on a belt, pendant, wrist, or ankle and can be located over a mile away.

2. *Companion Wanderer*, Pioneer Medical Systems, 37 Washington Street, Melrose, MA 02176. Tel. 617 662-2222. They carry a product that acts like an invisible fence. It can be used at home or away. Locator units are available.

3. *WanderGuard, Inc.*, P.O. Box 80238, Lincoln, NE 68501. Tel. 800 824-2996.

They make a full range of monitoring systems widely used in care facilities nationwide.

4. *Watch Mate System,* Instantel, Inc., Corporate offices: 362 Terry Fox Drive, Kanata, Ontario, Canada K2K 2P5. Tel. 613 592-4642. They also carry a full range of well-known monitoring systems.

In addition:

A wide variety of door and window alarms from hardware and electronics stores like Radio Shack are available. These can be glued or screwed to doors and windows, sounding an alarm when opened. Key and code models are available. Price: $15.00 and up.

Case Study: Assessment

The following case study illustrates the use of assessment tools to evaluate a patient's true ability to function, and the elimination of excess disability.

Mary

Mary is generally in a high moderate stage of dementia. She has lived in a large residential care facility for the elderly for about two weeks. Her daughter Anna stated on the behavior-rating instrument before placement that Mary dressed herself with some assistance every morning. In the residential care facility, however, Mary resists dressing and seems unable to carry out any of the steps with minimal help. Staff members evaluate her ability to dress herself at the "severe" level on the behavior-rating instrument, yet on a mental status test she tests at a high moderate level for both verbal comprehension and motor functioning ability.

The staff must reevaluate Mary or their own approaches and techniques. Perhaps Mary's daughter Anna inaccurately evaluated her mother's skills, but mental status test results tend to confirm Anna's rating. Perhaps the staff are approaching Mary incorrectly. Maybe she is still disoriented, depressed, or expressing anger over her placement.

In another conference, Anna says she still feels Mary can dress herself and carefully explains interaction techniques and cues she used to assist her mother with dressing. The staff now has a clearer picture of actual functioning level at home and insight into particular habits, likes, dislikes, and procedures the daughter used with Mary to get her to dress successfully. This new or revised information is recorded on the social history or in daily notes.

This information is then shared with all staff members. The staff may need to rethink their approaches. The dressing problem, interventions that the staff will be trying, and the ultimate goal are put into the care plan. Progress toward attaining the goal will be recorded in daily notes.

After a week or so of use of these *consistent positive* techniques to help with dressing, as written in the care plan, the staff will meet to evaluate progress. If progress is not satisfactory, another behavior rating, mental status test, and physical examination in conjunction with referral to the daily notes could be used to help reevaluate Mary's true ability to function. After evaluating the results as a team, the staff may need to revise the problem, goal, and approaches again on the care plan.

Case Study: Incorporating Activities in the Care Plan

The following case study illustrates emphasizing activity on the care plan as a goal and as an approach.

Martha

Martha is a seventy-year-old resident of a small, six-bed residential care facility and is diagnosed with multi-infarct dementia. She is very social and enjoys activities involving the opportunity to visit with others.

Her daughter, son-in-law, and their two teenage children live nearby and visit once a week. Their relationship is good.

Martha was a homemaker all of her life and enjoys food-preparation activities and crafts but will not participate in minor housekeeping chores enjoyed by other residents, such as folding laundry, sweeping the patio, or setting the table. She states very firmly that she did enough of that when she had a home of her own and does not want to participate anymore.

Martha's neurological symptoms, as measured on a mental status assessment and verified by day-to-day observations of the staff, are generally at the moderate stage, except for language ability and the use of motor skills (perception and organization of movement). These remain at a high level.

She is moderately impaired on the behavior-rating instrument, except in the areas of language, feeding herself, and dressing, which are in the light category. The staff rates Martha in the moderate stage for ability to perform household tasks because she refuses to participate. However, the staff thinks she could still perform them quite well if she wanted to. She is incontinent occasionally at night and she has recently had two episodes of urinary incontinence in the daytime, when no one reminded her to use the bathroom. These episodes have upset her greatly.

She has no behavior problems except that she is upset very easily if she is not dressed just right, if she is incontinent, or if she feels someone is ignoring her or has said something rude to her. There are two dementia patients who are often unaware of those around them or say inappropriate things to people. These residents are usually the ones who trigger her anger. She then remains upset for a long time afterward, though after a few minutes she does not know why she is angry.

Martha's health is fairly good, but the staff is concerned because she has some circulatory problems. She does not exercise much, and circulatory problems could be alleviated if she would get up and walk around more.

Martha's Patient Care Plan

PATIENT CARE PLAN

Patient's Name __Martha_____   Date_____

STAFF: Nursing: Soc Wk: Activities:

PROBLEM	GOALS	PLAN & APPROACHES	STAFF
I. Physical			
Sedentary, minor circulation problems.	Will move about more to improve circulation and general health	Will invite to join other residents (or friend/family) in all large motor activities, give one-on-one assistance in daily formal exercise, include walk on schedule daily, encourage/praise participation	Pers. Care Staff/ Actv.
Nighttime & occasional daytime incontinence	Will be continent 90% of the time at night and continent during the day	Will discourage excess liquids, remind her to use toilet before bed and between activities	
II. Psychosocial			
Very social. Enjoys a variety of activities but fairly sedentary (see Physical section)	Will continue to participate in activities, more large motor activity.	Will praise and encourage continued participation. Will emphasize large motor activity (see Physical section)	Pers. Care Staff/ Actv.
Is angered easily if ignored or if social contact is unpleasant	Will not be involved in confrontations with other residents.	Will not place near residents who anger her. Will be alert to potential problems and remove as necessary	
III. Family			
Family supportive. One friend visits	Family and friend will continue involvement	Keep family informed. Invite family and friend to activities	Soc. Serv./ Actv.

Monthly Review

Outcome: _____

Meeting Goals for Patients through Therapeutic Activities: The Stimulation of Retained Skills

Assess each individual's severity of neurological symptoms, level of functioning (emotional state, behavior problems, and ability to perform tasks of daily life), and remaining strengths and needs through the use of good formal assessment tools and documentation. Provide each patient with activities that maximize remaining skills, capitalize on strengths and needs, and minimize or avoid areas of weakness.

The caregiver must *always* remember that a person with dementia can not relearn. The goal of stimulation is to keep patients functioning at their true ability level for as long as possible (eliminating excess disability), not to help them relearn what they have already lost.

If a patient appears frustrated with an activity he or she has usually enjoyed, *drop it*. Perhaps the person is not feeling well, is distracted, or has declined in ability to function. Regardless of the reason, patients should *never* be pushed beyond their capacity. This can have severe consequences, including catastrophic reactions, behavior problems, drastic loss in self-esteem, and feelings of insecurity.

Appropriate stimulation of current level of:	*Is provided by involvement in:*
Memory (retention and retrieval)	Activities finished or related activities held over an extended period of time

Appropriate stimulation of current level of:	*Is provided by involvement in:*
Memory (retention and retrieval)	An activity theme followed for a day or several days Review of the day's successes and pleasures Use of simple calendars, clocks, daily activity schedules, and reminders of the day's events as cues throughout the day Caregivers can assist even more severely impaired patients by: • Giving frequent reminders of what an activity is and how to do it • Providing activities stimulating long-term memory. (Retention of long-term memory is actually a strength. See Handout IV:5.)
Language (receptive and expressive)	For mildly and moderately impaired patients: simple word games, conversation, discussion groups, following written instructions recipes and instructions, etc.), listening to, reading, or even composing simple stories and poems For all patients: active participation in conversations (may be very simple) and listening to others in conversation
Perceptual abilities, organization-of-movement abilities	Any large- or fine-motor activity Caregivers can assist by: • Using simple, easy-to-manage equipment • Using visual and tactile cues • Simplifying simple tasks even further for more severely impaired patients • Stressing activities familiar to patients, such as simplified versions of favorite active games (e.g., shuffleboard, bowling, and basketball) and daily living chores (e.g., housework and gardening).
Attention span, concentration	Almost all activities. This is done by engaging and reengaging the patient Activities involving constant active involvement are best. Example: A random game of catch is better than one in which patients take turns, because it requires their constant attention or patients will miss the ball

Appropriate stimulation of current level of:	*Is provided by involvement in:*
Abstract reasoning, judgment	For mildly and moderately impaired patients: any activity involving two or more interdependent steps—simple crafts and games, word games, reading, composing (with lots of assistance) simple poems or letters, some films, simple jigsaw puzzles, all familiar ADLs/IADLs, interrelating activities or associating them with holidays, times, or seasons, sorting projects
	For more severely impaired patients: the most basic associations or relationships are usually all that is retained. Most two-step tasks are too difficult
Appropriate emotional reaction, degree of reaction	Any activity that stimulates positive emotion but that does not overstimulate or that could be misinterpreted. (Example: A "Three Stooges" film may seem funny, but patients can easily misinterpret the slapstick as violent, harmful behavior.)
	Caregivers should watch for overstimulation, which can cause overreaction, and misinterpretation, which can cause inappropriate reaction. Patients readily react to emotional stimulation, and this is useful in activities. Positive use of emotion is a strength as well (Handout IV:5)

The Stimulation of Retained Strengths

Most dementia patients have certain strengths in common. Activities that stimulate these strengths will usually be the most successful.

Stimulation of:	*Is provided by involvement in:*
Use of habitual skills	Simplified versions of activities performed so many times throughout life that they can be executed without a great deal of conscious thought such as simplified ADLs/IADLs, social skills, and *very* simple versions of favorite games such as cards, dominoes, puzzles, horseshoes, golf. (Refer to Handouts V:14–24 for simplified activities.) It also includes talents like playing the piano, drawing, or sewing (but the caregiver must watch for frustration, because patients may be very aware they cannot perform the way they used to!)
Remote memory	Reminiscing activities such as reading or listening to especially chosen poems or stories, looking at old pictures, singing old familiar songs, playing familiar games, preparing favorite recipes
	Celebrating holidays and other special occasions

Stimulation of:	Is provided by involvement in:
Basic large- and fine-motor skills	Formal exercise, walks, simplified games involving large- and fine-motor movement, dancing, simple crafts
	Simplified ADLs/IADLs, including yard and household tasks
The basic senses	Almost all activities. Multiple cues; strong, pleasing sensations (bright, contrasting colors, pronounced textures); and variety are essential
Positive emotion	Time with visitors or pets, simple poetry and stories, old songs, simple jokes, anyone clowning around (as long as the patient interprets the actions correctly)
	The caregiver must remember to watch for over-stimulation (see Handout IV:4)
Positive use of perseveration	Any one-step activity that can be repeated over and over again, such as winding yarn or sweeping. (See list of one-step activities and rummaging activities in Handouts IV:9–10.)

Meeting Retained Needs

Most dementia patients have certain needs in common. Activities that meet these needs will usually be the most successful.

Maximization of:	*Is provided in all activities through:*
A sense of security	Use of good interaction techniques; use of the patient's name; smiles; a familiar, consistent schedule (but remember to still take advantage of spontaneous interests); staff familiarity with family names and patient history
Self-esteem	Encouraging patients to express opinions if they can, respecting their wishes and preferences
	Making sure an activity is appropriate (ensuring success) and meaningful to the person
	Helping in an activity when the patient has trouble (but not doing more than necessary)
	Switching to another activity if the patient is not enjoying it or is not succeeding
	Praising success, reminding the patient of successes, choosing activities and making their own choices within activities

Maximization of:	*Is provided in all activities through:*
Inclusion in the group	Repeating names, calling a patient's attention to people around them, leading group conversation, reminiscing and encouraging active participation, reminding patients of pleasant times they've had together, encouraging and praising teamwork, praising group successes

The Activities of Daily Living (ADLs) and Instrumental Activities of Daily Living (IADLs) in Daily Programming

The Activities of Daily Living (ADLs) are the most basic activities of day-to-day life. They are basic necessities and must be done daily or even several times daily for the maintenance of good health. A person with dementia should stay actively involved in these activities for as long as possible. As a patient's level of severity increases or if physical disabilities interfere, the activities should be simplified more and more, but the patient should continue to do at least part of an activity for as long as possible, in order to avoid excess disability. These activities are:

eating independently or with as little assistance as possible;

transferring into and out of bed, chairs, etc. (includes getting up and moving around during and between activities throughout the day);

mobility: walking indoors and out (includes vigorous daily walks whenever possible—the best way to combat wandering and pacing);

dressing independently or with as little assistance as possible (includes active participation in choosing clothing, pride in appearance);

grooming: brushing teeth and hair, shaving, applying makeup, pride in appearance;

bathing with as little assistance as possible;

toileting and continence care with as little assistance as possible.

The Instrumental Activities of Daily Living (IADLs) are generally more complex and less routine in nature than the ADLs. Dementia patients lose the ability to perform them alone very early in the disease. They are very meaningful in the everyday lives of all people, however, and it is important that patients continue to participate to some extent for as long as possible. They will probably need to be greatly simplified, or the patient may be able to participate in only some of the steps, not the entire activity. IADLs and suggestions of adaptations are:

Shopping	A patient could not shop alone but may enjoy planning and going shopping with others, continuing to help choose purchases, if possible. Planning and going on a shopping trip could be a theme for activities for several days
Meal preparation	Meal preparation is too complex for patients, but preparing one dish, with steps presented one at a time by the caregiver, is a wonderful activity
Housework	Individual, simplified housework activities are successful with most patients, as are simple yard and garden tasks
Laundry	Folding wash is a wonderful activity for the lowest-functioning patients. How about hanging wash out on an old-fashioned clothesline? Fresh air, motor stimulation, and a chance for reminiscing would all be benefits, along with fresh-smelling wash
Taking public transportation	This might be stressful for many patients, but it could be an enjoyable outing for confident, higher-functioning patients. Going for rides in a familiar automobile is fun for many patients, even very low-functioning people
Using the telephone	The telephone is often a problem for caregivers, but helping a patient to call relatives and friends can be both fun and an aid to short-term memory. Staff can turn it into a better activity by helping the patient list things he or she wants to talk about ahead of time, and then assisting with the call
Taking medication	The patient should *always* be monitored while taking medication and should *not* keep it in his or her possession. However, under direct supervision, the patient can continue to perform the steps himself or herself if he or she can do so without stress or difficulty

Money management   Ability to manage money is a skill lost early in dementia. The loss is upsetting to many patients, and
behavior problems involving money matters are
very common. However, it helps many patients feel
more secure and aids self-esteem to keep a purse or
wallet with them, carry small amounts of money,
and make small purchases with assistance on shopping trips

Planning and Implementing

a Therapeutic Activity

1. *When choosing an activity, consider the patient's:*

severity of neurological symptoms;
physical problems;
strengths and needs;
interests and preferences;
emotional state/behavior problems.

2. *Break the activity down into simple steps.* Each step should require the retention of only one concept at a time (one idea and action combination). High-functioning patients may be able to retain more.

3. *Make sure the environment is suitable and furniture is arranged properly.* Consider comfort, safety, grouping for easiest staff/patient interaction.

4. *Assemble all supplies before you begin.* Make sure the size and shape of any implements to be used are easy for the patient to handle. Have everything nearby for immediate use, but out of the patient's reach until needed (maybe even out of sight).

5. *Assess the patient immediately before beginning the activity.* Is this really the best time for the activity? Would another activity be better now? The caregiver must adapt the schedule to meet the patient's immediate needs.

6. *Invite the patient to join in.* Make sure the patient understands. Show her or him a sample or try saying, "Come with me, I'll show you." Be reassuring and positive. Remember, motivation must come from the caregiver.

7. *Be ready to start immediately.* Engage the patient right away.

8. *Present the first step.* Use multiple cues. Repeat instructions as necessary. Allow plenty of time before going on to the next step.

9. *Praise success; minimize any difficulties.* Help with any step if necessary, but stop doing so as soon as possible—do *not* do the activity for the patient. The patient should not be simply an observer. If it appears that observing is all that is possible, stop and reassess the situation. Is the activity too difficult? Does the patient dislike it? Simplify the activity further or provide an alternative activity.

HANDOUT IV:8

10. *If the patient seems to lose interest, engage and reengage her or him,* but watch for signs of stress; it is then time to stop. A patient may have to be engaged and reengaged many times. It is usually possible to stretch the patient's attention span to between thirty minutes and an hour in a well-designed, appropriate activity (and if attention span is not a severe problem for that patient).

11. *If the end result of an activity is a completed project, praise participation and success.* Remind the person later of the enjoyable time together.

Activities Based on Positive Use
of Perseveration

These activities consist of one basic step repeated over and over again. A few are really more than one step (sorting cards into blacks and reds or into suits, for example) but are so familiar to most patients that they are like one-step activities. Others can also be turned into "no-fail" rummaging activities. These are indicated with an asterisk (*) and are listed again in Handout IV:10.

FINE-MOTOR LEISURE ACTIVITIES:

Painting or coloring a large simple design with one color (a Christmas tree or Valentine heart, for example)
Cutting out basic shapes (hearts, strips, circles, squares, triangles)
Winding yarn, raffia, rope around a shape (around a cardboard strip to make a bracelet or napkin ring, for example) or into a ball
Unraveling and rolling the yarn in a clean old heavy knit sweater into balls for use in new projects
Spreading glue, sponge painting, or fingerpainting
Crushing, twisting, or rolling pieces of paper for various projects (to glue down for a collage, to string together for "flower" chains and necklaces)
Rolling balls, making coils, and flattening pieces of clay or play-dough for various projects
Sanding wood for cutting boards, children's blocks, large dominoes
Waxing sanded wood

Placing items onto a glue-covered surface for a collage
* Sorting or matching cards or dominoes
* Arranging flowers

LARGE-MOTOR LEISURE ACTIVITIES:

"Catch," either indoors (with a balloon ball) or outdoors (with a soft rubber ball)

"Volleyball" (tossing a ball back and forth over a net, a thick, brightly covered rope, or other easily visible barrier)

Tossing a parachute up and down (Physically fit patients may spontaneously want to run under it from one side to the other if it is a large one. Go with them for safety!)

Dancing

Walking

FINE-MOTOR DAILY LIVING ACTIVITIES:

Combing or brushing hair (the patient's own, another person's, a pet's fur)

Washing hands or face

Brushing teeth

Doing or getting neck rubs

* Folding wash (towels, pillowcases, or socks work best)

Ironing (with very careful supervision!)

* Washing dishes

* Drying dishes

* Putting away (in an easily accessible place) silverware, plates, cups

Rolling out dough

Kneading bread

Stirring

Stacking and sorting newspapers and magazines

* Folding letters and stuffing envelopes

Folding napkins

Dusting

LARGE-MOTOR DAILY LIVING ACTIVITIES:

Vacuuming or sweeping

Raking grass or leaves

Watering plants in the garden

Cleaning tabletops

Weeding (when discrimination between weeds and plants isn't absolutely necessary!)

Rummaging Boxes:

"No-Fail" Activities

There are no "correct" steps for a patient to follow in "no-fail" activities. The patient must simply be interested enough to enjoy handling the objects involved in some way.

It is easiest to keep supplies for each of the "no-fail" activities in separate boxes for quick and easy use. Use of these boxes is a good way to get support staff such as certified nurse assistants (CNAs) involved in leading patient activities. There are no specific instructions for the caregiver to follow, and patients can usually be engaged and stay engaged, at least for a while. Staff members can often even go on to other tasks or work with other patients nearby for a short while.

Patients often do not need to be provided with a reason to do rummaging activities. Simply seeing and touching the supplies is often enough to get them started. However, some patients may need to feel they are being useful. For example, it may help to ask a patient rummaging with the box of paper or plastic cups to "help stack the cups so that I can put them away." Higher-functioning patients will usually not respond well to "pretend work" activities, however, because they are aware that they are not truly helping, but they may still enjoy looking through collections of seashells, old postcards, and similar leisure activities "just for fun" or because it brings back pleasant memories.

"PRETEND WORK" DAILY LIVING SKILLS BOXES

Laundry: old towels or pillowcases are large enough for the patient to enjoy folding, but not too big or complicated for successful folding.

Socks to sort into pairs or just fold.

Keys and a variety of locks.

Various sizes of plastic jars and lids to match together.

Plastic eating utensils and silverware bins to sort them in.

Dishwashing: a large dishpan, sponge, adult size plastic dishes, mild soap, and plenty of towels to mop up spills.

Plastic or large sturdy paper cups and plates to stack and sort (different sizes and colors could be stacked together).

LEISURE-TIME BOXES

Rickrack, laces, and ribbon (fairly short pieces for safety reasons) to sort and roll.

Yarn to wind into balls. Pieces of many different colors, all several feet in length, can be wound together and placed in the box. The patient can then wind them into small individual balls.

Bows.

Large buttons to sort. Small ones grouped by size and color and fastened securely to small loops of rope or elastic to avoid swallowing by patients may be OK.

Plastic vases and artificial flowers to arrange. Wrap stems to avoid sharp points.

Blocks of wood that "need" sanding and sandpaper.

Large nuts and bolts to screw together.

Letters to fold and envelopes to stuff (get discards from the business office).

Colorful fabric squares of different textures to lay out and arrange in "quilt" designs.

Fairly large felt or fabric shapes to arrange into unusual designs and pictures (these could be various geometric shapes, birds, trees, animals, flowers).

Colorful scarves.

Old jewelry (check for loose stones and take backs off of pins).

Greeting cards.

Large colored pictures (from calendars) mounted on cardboard.

Photos.

Dominoes to lay out in designs and sort.

Playing cards to lay out and sort.

COLLECTIBLES BOXES

Seashells (but not tiny ones)

Postcards

Miniature toy cars, boats, trains

Small plastic toy animals
Small dolls
Small stuffed animals

THEME BOXES

HANDOUT IV:10

Items for individual holidays: Christmas, Halloween, Easter, Valentine's Day, patriotic items (flags, armed services insignia, hats) for Memorial Day, Armed Services Day, and Independence Day.

Vacation boxes: things to take camping, to the shore, from particular countries.

Childhood memories (toys, pictures of children and children and their parents, items of clothing children or babies wear).

Pets (stuffed animals, pictures, collars and leashes, food dishes).

Types of clothing popular when they were young (pictures and actual items).

Items having to do with any good topic for reminiscing will work. Use your imagination!

Suggested Resources: Activities

for Persons with Dementia

Books

Cohen, Pat Stacey, and Sincox, Rochelle. 1986. *Adapting the Adult Day Care Environment for Older Adults with Dementia.* Winnetka, Ill.: Illinois Department of Aging.

Dowling, James R. 1995. *Keeping Busy: A Handbook of Activities for Persons with Dementia.* Baltimore: Johns Hopkins University Press.

Nissenboim, Silvia, and Vroman, Christine. 1989. *Interactions by Design: The Positive Interactions Program for Persons with Alzheimer's Disease and Related Disorders.* St. Louis: Geri-Active Consultants.

Sheridan, Carmel. 1987. *Failure-Free Activities for the Alzheimer's Patient: A Guidebook for Caregivers.* San Francisco, Calif.: Cottage Books.

Thews, Vikki; Reaves, Antonia; and Henry, Rona, eds. 1993. *Now What?: A Handbook of Activities for Adult Day Programs.* Winston-Salem, N.C.: Bowman Gray School of Medicine, Wake Forest University.

Zgola, J. 1987. *Doing Things: A Guide to Programing Activities for Persons with Alzheimer's Disease and Related Disorders.* Baltimore: Johns Hopkins University Press.

Mail-Order Catalogs

Bifolkal Productions, Inc.
809 Williamson Street
Madison, WI 53703
Phone: 800 568-5357; 608 251-2818

Slide presentation kits for reminiscing with audiotapes and props to use for additional sensory awareness. The kits are not specifically designed for persons with dementia, but they work very well.

Sensibilities: Activities for the Cognitively Impaired Older Adult
Geriatric Educational Consultants
P.O. Box 1178
Holmes Beach, FL 34218
Phone: 941 778-7050

Activity products specifically designed for those with dementia.

Hammatt Senior Products
1 Sportime Way
Atlanta, GA 30340
Phone: 800 428-5127

Many suitable activity supplies.

Medical and Activity Sales Catalog
2869 Bondesson, P.O. Box 12476
Omaha, NE 68112
Phone: 800 541-9152; 402 457-3500

Many products are suitable for persons with dementia but are not labeled as such. The buyer must choose carefully.

S&S Arts and Crafts
75 Mill Street, P.O. Box 513
Colchester, CT 06415
Phone: 800 243-9232

The catalog uses a cognitive-level rating system for some of the activity kits. Other kits and supplies can be adapted for use with dementia patients or are at least a good source of ideas.

List of Suggested Activities

for Persons with Dementia

The activities listed below can be adapted for use in carrying out many of the themes listed in "Daily and Weekly Themes for Use in Program Planning" (Handout V:8). They are all based on activities commonly enjoyed by cognitively normal older adults but can be adapted to consist of no more than a few simple steps.

Some patients may be able to engage independently in those activities with an asterisk (") once the caregiver helps them to begin. These have only one step and are based on "positive use of perseveration" or are "no-fail" (also see Module IV).

Service Projects

Service projects stimulate self-esteem, awareness of the group (the community), and a sense of belonging.

1. Do things to enhance and maintain the facility: Make puzzles, cutting boards, wall decorations, checkerboards, photo albums, napkin rings and placemats, pillows; prepare a garden, flower arrangements, invitations, a calendar board; stuff envelopes; wash windows; vacuum; scrub tables; dust; sweep; rake leaves.

2. Many churches, synagogues, and other religious and service organizations have ongoing service projects for those in need in the United States and around the world. Cutting fabric squares and tearing and *rolling bandages for use in

sewing classes and in hospitals around the world has been successful at our centers.

3. Make pine cone bird feeders and donate them to parks.

4. Make toys for the animals at the Humane Society. *Some patients can braid yarn toys independently.

5. Make giant dominoes, puzzles, and blocks (or refinish old blocks) for preschools.

6. *Stuff envelopes for any organization.

7. Design and make thank-you notes.

8. Make projects for local religious organizations, schools, and hospitals: centerpieces, tray and table decorations, etc.

9. Check around your community and work with a variety of local organizations.

Active Games

Active games stimulate large- and fine-motor skills, inclusion in and interaction with a group, habitual skills, reasoning, and memory.

Basketball: Throw a ball in a basket; use teams and give points.

Miniature golf or putting practice: Make up your own version, using soft, larger balls and easy-to-hit target holes.

Volleyball: Indoors, seated, use a balloon ball. Outdoors, standing (if safe) or seated, use a large, light rubber ball.

"Football": Kick a ball over a "goal"; use teams and give points.

Simplified shuffleboard.

"Soccer" (seated). Similar to football.

Horseshoes: Adult plastic versions—still hard, be careful!

Weighted lawn darts (*not* sharp, pointed darts).

Dartboard game using plastic darts.

Parachute toss—many variations.

Frisbee toss, using a soft frisbee.

*Dancing: twosomes, group, "square dancing."

Beanbag toss (many varieties).

Squirt gun games (at targets, not at each other!).

Knocking down a tin can tower with a rubber ball.

Pitching pennies.

Tossing cards in a hat.

*Balloon ball, in a circle (background music can set the mood).

*Tossing a rubber playground ball to each other: Outdoors, standing or seated in a circle.

Discussion Groups and Word Games

Discussion groups and word games stimulate remote memory, language skills, positive use of emotion, inclusion in a group, and a sense of security. *Note:* Discussion groups and word games tie in well with various themes. Word games are usually done on a whiteboard.

List games: List words starting with each letter of the alphabet. All words relate to a chosen topic. For example, discuss autumn. Then patients list all the words that they can think of with associations to autumn.

Other word games:

Hidden word games
Simple crossword puzzles
"Fill in the blanks" word games
Trivia
Spelling bees
Definitions games
Listening and responding to jokes
Listening to short stories and poetry

Composing letters and poetry
Watching and discussing a film or slides (choose carefully!)
Watching and listening to a demonstration (handle objects too, if possible) and *short* talk, any special visitor

Tabletop Games

Tabletop games stimulate fine-motor and some large-motor skills, group interaction, inclusion in a group, reasoning, and memory.

Marble games
Tabletop ball games: Just rolling a ball to each other around a table is fun; music in the background sets the mood
Pitching pennies
Tabletop "hockey"
Tabletop pinball
Tabletop shuffleboard, using beanbags or small balls

Simplified dominoes
Simplified card games
Adult (yet simple) board games
Puzzles: Adult-looking, with 2 to 20 pieces. Try having patients make their own—it's a good craft project. (Exception to the 20-piece rule: U.S. puzzles are great!)

Performing Activities of Daily Living

Performing ADLs stimulates self-esteem, identity, large- and fine-motor skills, remote memory, ability to perform habitual skills, and the basic senses.

Nail care
Applying makeup

Combing hair
Dressing, choosing accessories, etc.

Caring for a pet

Sewing on buttons, hems, etc. (for
　high-functioning patients)

Setting the table

Cleaning up after eating

*Washing or drying dishes

*Dusting

Making beds

*Sweeping

*Raking

*Vacuuming

Preparing food

Crafts

Crafts stimulate receptive language ability, reasoning and judgment, fine-motor coordination, dexterity, and self-esteem, and provide a chance to make independent choices.

Braided cloth wreaths (*braiding or twisting the cloth).

Covered and wrapped containers and jewelry: "leather look" (tape covered), tissue paper collage, *wrapped with yarn or raffia squares, etc. (*patients enjoy arranging the shapes).

Mosaic plaques, trivets, and coasters: ceramic tile, bean, or fabric.

Bottles of layered colored sand.

*Coloring: *Adult* books are available (don't use children's!); enlarge designs if too small and complex.

*Making stationery or wall decorations, placemats: coloring, pasting, use dried flowers, leaf prints, negative printing.

Tissue paper roses.

Potpourri hoops and braided wall hangings.

Pompom animals.

"Batik" tissue paper for wall hangings or wrapping paper: Fold tissue paper several different ways, dip corners in different colors of food coloring. Dry, unwrap carefully. Beautiful!

Dough ornaments.

Clay beads.

Covering Styrofoam shapes: Use a variety of coverings (small, torn pieces of paper or fabric, dried flowers), anchored in place using brass fasteners or large-headed pins (use with care) to make wreaths, Christmas trees, etc.

Cardboard as a base for wreaths or other decoration: Glue on different coverings—pine cones, dried flowers, rolled paper balls.

*Free-form watercolor and acrylic painting: Makes beautiful stationery, book covers, placemats, and wall hangings when cut and glued on plain paper border backgrounds.

*Threading beads for necklaces and decorations.

*Making magazine paper beads for necklaces: Glue and roll long triangles of paper (approximately 1″ by 3″). String as beads.

*Cutting shapes from construction paper: Staple together to make paper chains for decorating the room. Paper valentine hearts are a favorite.

Christmas tree ornaments: pine cones (paint on glue, sprinkle with glitter); folded paper fan ornaments; cut shapes from old Christmas cards, tie on a ribbon to hang; projects using protective adhesive coatings such as Mod-podge (calendars or pictures onto decorative backings, dried flower arrangements on backings, containers) (*brushing modpodge under and over shapes being anchored).

Tie dying (needs lots of volunteers, but fun).

Coloring stencils.

Woodworking (*sanding or rubbing in paste wax can be independent for short periods of time): dominoes, blocks, cutting boards, photo albums, simple stools, trays, photo blocks, hammering nails into wood, wooden boats and race cars for races (invite Boy or Girl Scouts, other children's clubs, host races).

Quiet "Wind Down" or "No-Fail" Activities

Quiet "wind down" or "no-fail" activities provide a chance for patients to relax and be free of more intense cognitive demands; they are calming in stressful situations or if patients are experiencing Sundowner syndrome. They are ideal for low-functioning patients.

Rolling a ball back and forth to each other on a tabletop

Talking

Sing-along

*Listening to music

*Moving to music

*Walking

Getting neck rubs

*Looking at magazines or large pictures

*Looking at photos

*Rummaging (see Module IV): laundry, old cards and photos, fabrics, jewelry, almost any objects that are safe and of interest to the patient

*Sorting, stacking activities: blocks, Jenga game, screws, nuts and bolts, buttons; arranging wooden, paper, felt, or other fabric shapes on a light-colored surface

*Sanding wood

*Winding yarn

*Unraveling an old sweater

*Shelling peas, peanuts, cracking walnuts (careful!)

Planning and Leading Successful Group Activities

Step 1: Choosing and Planning the Activity

Can this activity be adapted for successful use by a particular patient group?

Consider the interests, strengths, weaknesses, and general functioning level of potential participants.

Think about staff members to lead the activity. Choose those who will be the most confident and who will enjoy leading it.

Where should the activity take place? How should the room or space be arranged? Plan the placement of furniture, supplies, and the seating of patients.

Break the activity down into simple steps, each step requiring one idea and action not based on previous steps.

"Walk through" steps to make sure they are appropriate. Determine the amount of time needed. What time of day would be best?

In the "walk through," think about the supplies and tools. Will patients be able to handle them well? If not, can they be adapted?

If the activity still seems like a good idea, purchase and assemble supplies.

Make a sample or provide other cues to aid patients' comprehension.

Step 2: Getting the Activity Started

Reassess the patients for the group. Should some patients be added or deleted? Will some participants have special needs today (more simplification, seating away from other participants, etc.)?

Is this time *really* OK for this activity? Be flexible!

Make sure there is enough time. Don't rush!

Set up the space. Make sure there are no distractions, no discomforts, such as glare, wind, etc.

Assemble *all* supplies, in *your* reach, but out of reach of patients.

Invite the patients *one at a time.*

Use eye contact, touch, a warm smile. Getting them there takes time. Show them samples, supplies, or other types of cues or point to the activity area to make sure they understand.

Have one staff member keep bringing in patients while another staff person engages those who are already there.

Begin as soon as possible.

Step 3: Doing the Activity

The staff should create a positive atmosphere with their enthusiasm, facial expressions, tone of voice, and body language.

Present the first step very simply. Make sure that *only* supplies for this step are out in front of the patient.

Keep a sample on display if it is a craft. Repeat the goal.

Repeat instructions slowly and patiently.

Allow plenty of time for the step!

Engage and reengage as necessary.

Watch for patients losing attention, recall their attention before they actually leave.

Spend time with *each patient.* Get and maintain eye contact with each one.

Don't play favorites. Even if one person needs more help, spend time with all.

Go on to the next step when the majority of the patients are ready. Remove all supplies from the previous step.

Praise successes! Minimize failures.

Step in and help as necessary, but step out again as soon as patients can proceed successfully on their own.

Patient success is *the primary goal.* If a goal is a final product or result, encourage completion but don't push.

Step 4: After the Activity

Praise participation. Don't point out mistakes.

If there is a final *successful* product, display it, reminding patients of the activity.

Thank each patient for participating.

Remind all patients of successful, pleasant activities afterward.

Memories of pleasant times and success give life meaning. Patients cannot remember recent good times all on their own. Staff members must remind and reinforce.

Cue Card: A Short Guide to Successful Group Activities

Put these quick references on a 5" × 7" card and keep it handy for a cue to implementation of activities. Remember, these are *only* the main points!

FRONT OF CARD:

Planning and Implementing Activities

Before the activity:

Group patients by interests and strengths.

Plan for a small group, allowing for individual attention.

Tailor an activity for the group. It must be adult, consist of between one and four steps (depending on the group's functioning level), and be geared for patient success.

Simplify implements and supplies for maximum success.

Arrange the room or area for maximum success.

Arrange all supplies within *your* reach, out of patients' reach.

Allow plenty of time.

Reassess before starting: Is it right for each patient right now?

During the activity:

Engage each patient as soon as he or she arrives.

Try to ensure that patients understand the concept: Display a craft sample or explain *very simply* the final result; repeat often.

Put supplies for *only* one step at a time within patients' reach.

Demonstrate and repeat *simple* instructions for each step often.

Praise success and minimize mistakes.

Quickly reengage patients who start to lose attention.

Encourage and praise completion, but don't push.

After the activity:

Thank them; remind them of and praise positive results!

HANDOUT V:4

Instructions for Various
Group Activities

Dominoes

GOALS To stimulate remote memory, use of fine-motor skills, dexterity, feelings of inclusion in a group, and self-esteem; and to maximize reasoning, perceptual, and organization-of-movement skills.

Functioning level of participants: The game is appropriate for moderately impaired and higher-functioning patients any time of the day. It is not appropriate for those with very short attention spans, since patients must take turns.

Size of group: One staff person can play with two to six patients. If more play, it is a long wait between turns.

Equipment and supplies needed: One set of dominoes, preferably color coded. Oversized dominoes are useful for visually impaired patients. (Look in adult activity catalogs [see Handout V:1]. Or make them—it is a good craft project.) A small tray is also needed.

Arrangement of space and furniture; positioning of staff and patients: The table should not be too large. Patients should sit in close to the table, with the middle of the table within easy reach. The staff member should position him or herself at the table so that all patients' dominoes are within easy reach. Assistance may be needed.

Steps: The object of the game is for players to get rid of all their dominoes by matching them end to end with those already out in play on the table. The winner is the first person out of dominoes.

1. Place all dominoes face down in the middle of the table on the tray (patients enjoy doing this). Patients can take turns drawing dominoes. The person choosing the highest double during the first draw starts play. If no double is drawn, they choose again until one is drawn. Or, the person to the left of the leader starts (this is easier). Each patient draws seven dominoes and turns them face up in front of them. (Leader may have to cue counting them out and turning them over. If they are placed slightly apart, dots are easier to distinguish.)

2. The extra dominoes—the "bone pile"—should be left on the tray to one side. (If patients must draw from the bone pile, the tray can be moved close to them so they can draw their own.)

3. The person to start play places any of his or her dominoes face up in the middle of the table.

4. The next person must match one end of the domino in the middle of the table. The leader may have to point out which domino matches, covering up one side of the domino and pointing out the dots that match. (Patients get the two sides of dots confused, and this is why color-coded dominoes are useful.) If the person doesn't have a matching domino, he or she must draw from the bone pile until he or she gets one. If the bone pile has been used up, the person must skip a turn.

5. Play continues around the table until someone is out of dominoes and wins. Players may match at either end of the domino chain. If the string gets so long that players can't reach the ends, turn and start back, creating a zigzag effect.

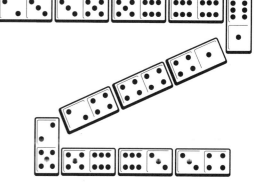

Adaptations: For higher-functioning patients, build out at the sides on doubles (this is too confusing for most patients). Lower-functioning patients enjoy just handling and arranging the dominoes.

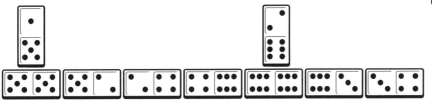

Tabletop Pinball

GOALS To stimulate the use of fine-motor skills and dexterity and feelings of self-esteem and inclusion in a group, and to maximize perceptual and organization-of-movement skills and attention span.

Functioning level of participants: The game is appropriate for mildly impaired to low second-stage patients. It keeps the interest of large groups of patients even in late afternoon.

Size of group: One leader and two to seven patients can play.

Equipment and supplies needed: Three 2″ brightly colored rubber or golf balls (must contrast in color to tabletop for visibility), masking tape, black marker pen, plastic bowl large enough to hold three balls, and enough disposable coffee cups so that, when almost touching side to side, they could line the short end of a long table. They should be cut and numbered as follows:

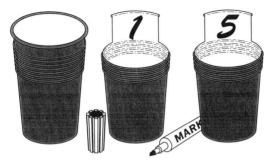

Arrangement of space and furniture; positioning of staff and patients: Allow at least ten minutes to prepare. It takes a while to tape the cups to the table edge. A table at least five feet long or two smaller square or rectangular tables placed end to end are needed (they must be level and meet evenly). Tape the cups side by side along one short end of the table, with numbers on the "tabs" of the cups as shown above. For maximum patient success, don't leave spaces between cups.

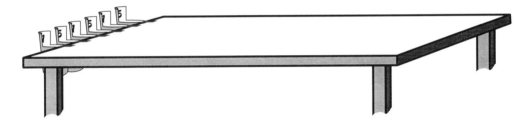

Place chairs for participants around three sides of the table. Two participants can be seated at each of the long sides, one participant at each corner, and one participant at the end away from the cups. The group leader should sit behind the cups. (It is important for the leader to sit, to maintain eye contact with the participants, to demonstrate, and to roll balls back to the participants.) Lower-functioning, visually impaired, or physically weaker participants should sit at the long sides of the table closest to the cups, for easy assistance from the leader. (No one should be seated within two feet of the cups or the game will be too easy—balls could just be dropped into the cups.)

Process: The object of the game is for participants to roll all three balls into cups. If a ball goes off the table, the turn can be repeated. If it lands between cups, the score is 0. The score for a turn is the total of the numbers on the cups holding balls.

The leader hands the container of balls to the first player and instructs him or her to roll one ball into the cups. The leader may have to hand each ball to some players, tap the cups, place the player's hand correctly, etc. To help the player visualize the score, the leader should leave the balls in the cups till the turn is over.

The player with the highest score after a set time wins.

HANDOUT V:5

The List Game

The following is adapted from Michele M. Nolta, "A to Z Game," Recreation Therapy Consultants, San Diego (phone: 619 546-9003).

GOALS Stimulation of remote memory, feelings of self-esteem, and inclusion in a group; maximization of reasoning and language ability.

Functioning level of participants: It is appropriate for mildly impaired to second-stage patients who retain language skills.

Size of group: One leader, three to ten patients. A second staff member to prompt, assist, reengage more impaired patients would be useful.

Equipment and supplies needed: A whiteboard and dark marker. Visual and tactile props related to the theme are useful.

Arrangement of space and furniture; positioning of staff and patients: The leader should be positioned by the whiteboard. Patients should be seated close enough to stay engaged and see the board well, no farther than ten feet away from the leader. Position a second staff person with lower-functioning participants or those with short attention spans.

Process: Choose a theme of interest to patients and think of a variety of words and word associations related to the theme. (For example, "Winter Fun" conjures up thoughts of snow, sleds, snowmen, mittens, scarves, fires in the fireplace, etc., for those from cold climates.) Write the theme at the top of the board and the letters of the alphabet in two columns. The object of the activity is for participants to think of as many words related to the theme as they can, starting with as many letters of the alphabet as possible. As patients think of a word, write it under the correct letter of the alphabet on the board.

1. Set the mood by talking about the theme subject a little. (Use props if available.)
2. Tell the group the idea of the game is to think of words having to do with the theme. Give definitions of words to draw out ideas. (For example, using the theme given above, "What do you call the piece of cloth that you wrap around your neck when it is cold?")
3. Encourage quiet group members. Require only "yes" and "no" responses from lower-functioning participants. (For example, you know a patient used to love to ice skate. Say: "Joe, I understand you used to love to skate in winter. Is that right?")

Basketball

GOALS To stimulate large-motor skills, balance, muscle control, sense of inclusion in a group, and self-esteem; and to maximize perceptual and appropriate organization-of-movement skills.

Functioning level of participants: The game is appropriate for higher-functioning and moderately impaired patients. Those with short attention spans may wander off as patients take turns.

Size of group: One leader can play with up to fourteen patients.

Equipment and supplies needed: Whiteboard and marker for score keeping, team logos to help team members have fun, a ten- to twelve-inch play ball, and a *deep* basket or box (to keep the ball from bouncing out) or low basketball net. (Dementia patients have trouble looking up and throwing a ball into a net above eye level. Don't use a child's net, however. Look in adult activity catalogs [see Handout V:1] or mount a regular net no higher than six feet off the ground.)

Arrangement of space and furniture; positioning of staff and patients: Use a large open area, preferably outdoors. Arrange chairs and spaces for wheelchairs in two parallel rows ten feet apart. The net should be about six feet beyond one end of the rows.

Steps: Each row of patients is a team. Higher-functioning patients may enjoy choosing team names and could wear a team logo on their shirts to reinforce the team concept and spirit. (Making logos could be a craft project as part of a basketball theme before play.) Team names are written on the board. The score for each team is kept underneath. The first team to reach twenty-one points wins.

1. The first patients in each row can flip a coin to choose which team starts.
2. Each player takes two throws at each turn. Play alternates between teams and proceeds from one end of each row. Each patient should stand, or sit if necessary, about six feet back from the basket and throw the ball in. (Getting up and moving about provides some of the large-motor stimulation of the game. Watching a player get up and throw adds more visual stimulation and opportunity for group interaction for those waiting for a turn.)
3. The game ends when one team reaches twenty-one points. The leader can keep the team spirit lively by calling out team scores occasionally, etc.

ADAPTATIONS: For lower-functioning patients, keep score for individuals, not teams. Or, patients just enjoy making baskets. Move the basket lower and closer.

Instructions for Various Card Games

"Match It!"

GOALS To stimulate remote memory, use of fine-motor skills, dexterity, feelings of inclusion in a group, and self-esteem; and to maximize attention span and perceptual skills.

Functioning level of participants: The game is appropriate for moderately impaired and high-functioning patients and has successfully kept patients' attention even in late afternoon.

Size of group: One staff person can play with three to eight patients.

Equipment and supplies needed: Two decks of cards are needed. Some patients may respond better to large-print cards. Others don't respond as well to these because they are unfamiliar.

Arrangement of space and furniture; positioning of staff and patients: The table can be round, square, or rectangular, but not too large. Patients should sit close to the table, with the middle of the table within easy reach. Staff members should position themselves at the table so that all patients' cards are within easy reach, since assistance may be needed.

Steps: The object of the game is for participants to get rid of all cards by discarding those that match those held by the leader. The winner is the first person out of cards.

1. Deal out all cards from one deck (a patient may be able to do this). Each

patient receives the same number of cards, but use as much of the deck as possible. The leader keeps unused cards for reference.

2. Patients place their cards face up in front of them so staff members can assist more easily. They should place cards of the same suit together for easier identification (with assistance as needed).

3. The leader holds the other deck of cards. The leader then holds up one card from the deck, shows the card to everyone, and repeats the suit and number several times, to ensure that all participants understand.

4. The patient with the matching card places it face down in the middle of the table (so that the patient does not mix discards with the remaining cards). Patients may need cuing each time. Some patients need tactile assistance as well, but the leader should assist as little as possible. Picking up and moving the cards about provides the fine-motor stimulation of the activity.

5. The leader must frequently remind participants of the purpose of the game and point out which players have the fewest cards. This stimulates excitement, group interaction skills, and the self-esteem of the winner.

Sequences

GOALS To stimulate remote memory, use of fine-motor skills, dexterity, feelings of inclusion in a group, and self-esteem; and to maximize perceptual skills and attention span.

Functioning level of participants: The game is appropriate for moderately impaired patients (higher-functioning patients usually lose interest).

Size of group: One leader and two to six patients can play.

Equipment and supplies needed: One deck of cards.

Arrangement of space and furniture; positioning of staff and patients: Same as for "Match It!"

Steps: The object of the game is to discard all cards. This is done by discarding all cards to the center of the table by suits, in the order of smallest value to largest. The first person out of cards is the winner.

1. Deal out all cards from the deck (a patient may be able to do this). Give each patient the same number of cards, but use as much of the deck as possible. The leader keeps unused cards for reference.

2. Participants place their cards face up in front of them so staff members can assist more easily. Cards of the same suit can be placed together for easier identification.

3. The leader asks the person to his or her left to start. The person can start if he or she has a "2" of any suit. If the person doesn't have a "2," play

proceeds on around to the left until someone does. The "2" is placed face up in the middle of the table.

4. The person with the next card of that suit plays next. The discards are placed side by side in sequence in the middle of the table (this is a visual cue to help patients see which card should be discarded next). Play proceeds until all cards of that suit are discarded in order.

5. The person to the left of the player with the last card of the suit must start the discard of a new suit by placing a "2" in the middle of the table (remove all of the cards of the first suit to avoid confusion). Play then proceeds as in steps 3 and 4 above for each suit.

6. The first person out of cards is the winner. Or, play can proceed until all cards are out in order. (Patients out of cards will lose interest, however.)

Cards for Low-Functioning Patients

GOALS To maximize remaining level of awareness, long-term memory, and perceptual and organization-of-movement skills.

Functioning level of participants: These activities are appropriate for residents in the low second stage and even some in the third stage.

(Higher-functioning patients lose interest.)

Size of group: One staff person can assist one to four patients.

Equipment and supplies needed: One to several decks of cards.

Arrangement of space and furniture; positioning of staff and patients: Same as for "Match It!"

Process: Three different basic card activities are given below.

Activities 2 and 3 are not really games, because there are no winners or losers.

Card activity 1: Use two decks. Play a simplified version of "Match It!" The leader displays cards from only *one* full suit, however. Patients can discard *all* cards they have with the same value as the leader's.

Card activity 2: Assist patients in sorting cards into suits or just into colors. Some patients may be able to work together, or each patient can have a deck.

Card activity 3: The leader can just use verbal and tactile cues to get patients to handle and move cards about. This is all that some very-low-functioning patients are able to do.

What Can You Do about Patients
Who Won't Participate?

The New Patient

New patients or residents need a lot of time and care.

1. Immediately become familiar with the person's history and show the person your interest. Since the patient has short-term memory loss, you and the rest of the staff may really be strangers, even if you have met before. Everything you do must reassure the person that you know something about him or her, are friendly, and can be trusted. Positive body language and facial expression is vital, especially if the patient can no longer communicate verbally.
   a. Spend extra time with them or assign a staff person to do so.
   b. During each visit, reinforce that you are a friend. Reintroduce yourself, mention your previous visits. Use positive tactile and visual cues.
   c. Each time you visit, let the person know you already know and care about him or her.
   d. All staff members should use a consistent, positive approach.
2. Remind the person of and reinforce positive experiences in the new surroundings. The home the person left is what is real and familiar to him or her. The person misses it. Due to the short-term memory loss, the person does not remember all the new people and things he or she is now experiencing. It will take the person a long time and a lot of positive reinforce-

ment from you and other staff members to feel comfortable in the new surroundings.

   a. Create and then reinforce lots of positive experiences.

   b. Remind the person of pleasant visits with other patients often. Reintroduce them each time.

   c. Remind the person of enjoyable times and activities that have occurred so far. Repeat them.

   d. Introduce further changes in routine, surroundings, or activities very gradually. Go slow!

The Reluctant Patient

The patient who is reluctant to join in needs the same attention as the new patient. Your goal with this type of person should be small, gradual improvements. Document all efforts to gain the person's involvement and any small successes.

All patients who are still aware to some degree should be involved in some activities daily. *Minimal* daily involvement in activities for all but the lowest-functioning patients should include:

1. positive interaction with the staff several times daily;
2. some active involvement in ADLs;
3. some positive involvement with other patients and group activities;
4. Some involvement in therapeutic activity other than routine ADLs.

To get a reluctant participant more involved:

1. Know the person. Start by suggesting activities that you feel would interest the person most.
2. Overcome language barriers.
   a. When inviting the person to join, say, "let me show you something" or "keep me company." Do not give a long explanation of the activity. Use tactile and visual cues.
   b. At the activity, make sure the person understands it. Use gestures, visual cues, samples.
3. Ease the person's fears.
   a. The person may be afraid to leave a familiar location. Reassure the person that you are taking him or her to a pleasant place, that the person has been there before, and that you will stay with the person and take him or her back to his or her room (always follow through).
   b. The person may be afraid he or she will fail. Reassure the person that he or she can do it, that you will help, or that the person can "just

watch" (usually "watchers" gradually participate if urged again *very gently* once the activity begins).

4. Remember that the person is an adult used to making his or her own decisions. The person may be refusing to participate as a way of maintaining self-esteem and freedom of choice.

   a. Request the person's company. It should not sound like an order.

   b. Some patients may feel better if they come when they feel like it, not when you first invite them. If they are seated where they can see the activity or if you come back and remind them later, they may join in. If they can't see the activity going on or they are not reminded later, they will forget all about it. (You may want to move the activity to a spot near them if they refuse to move, maybe even close enough so they can join in without moving.)

   c. If it is an activity that a patient can safely do alone, leave the supplies beside the person and say you could really use the help. The person may begin when you are gone. Doing an activity when the person feels like it, not when you tell him or her to, can help the person preserve self-esteem.

   d. Provide choices.

   e. Ask for the person's help with another participant or with the activity. Say you would like the person's company, need a partner, or just can't proceed without another participant. Make sure to thank the person afterward. These approaches can be real self-esteem builders.

Daily and Weekly Themes for Use

in Program Planning

Holidays.

The seasons.

Special entertainment: Preparing for a party.

Any special visit: A demonstration, or slides and a very short "lecture," or children's visit. Build a day or two around the specific topic to be presented.

"Home by the fire": Indoor, at-home-type activities for midwinter.

Presidents.

Anniversaries of statehood for various states.

Pets.

Animals of various types: Desert animals, animals of a specific country or climate, marine animals, imaginary trips to the zoo.

Travel: Armchair visits to Africa (emphasize safari or culture), Korea, Japan, Germany (Oktoberfest), England, Ireland (St. Patrick's Day), China (Chinese New Year), Mexico (Cinco De Mayo), Italy, Russia, Alaska, Hawaii, the southern United States, the southwestern United States (western and American Indian themes), and California are all popular. Patients, families, and staff members can participate by sharing mementoes and slides.

Specific types of trips: Camping, fishing, hiking, to the mountains, to the seashore, cruises, and reminiscing about favorite trips are all popular.

Special types of clothing: Hat Day and Dress-Up Day (around Easter), old-fashioned clothing, Tee Shirt Day, western.

Recognition of volunteers.

Reminiscing:

- "When we were young": Things they did as children in various seasons and on holidays, favorite books and nursery rhymes, first day of school, favorite games and toys, favorite foods, memories of Mother and Father, relationships with siblings, and pets.
- Young adulthood: Memories of the war years, the Depression, first date, first car, first job, wedding, times with their young children.
- Places and things: Old cars, furniture and appliances they or their parents used, clothing, the farm, their home city in the past, places they've lived.

"Lazy days of summer": Silly "goof-off" activities, bubble blowing, soaking their feet, playing with sand, "tee-shirt day," telling knock-knock jokes.

County fairs.

Harvest time.

Arts and crafts shows or "Be an Artist Week."

Hobby shows.

The circus.

Back to school.

Apple harvest.

Special sporting events: Hold similar activities when major local, national, or international events are taking place: the Olympics, golf tournaments, auto and horse races, bowling tournaments, football, basketball, baseball, hockey.

Local festivals: Auto shows, "tall ships" festivals, Centennial and Old Town festivals, rodeos.

Holidays: Holidays can be emphasized for two or three weeks by planning themes around the preparation for a very special parties or for their own celebrations at home.

- Halloween: For a party, several days each: Preparing treats, decorating, simple costume ideas.
- Thanksgiving: For a special lunch or dinner to which families are invited, several days each: Preparing invitations, preparing food, decorating, community service projects.
- Christmas: For parties at the facility and for family get-togethers, several days each: Making and sending Christmas cards, preparing special Christmas service projects, decorating, preparing refreshments and decorations for parties, making and wrapping gifts for families.

Schedule of the Day

Date: _____

Time	Activity and Instructions	Staff Responsible

Effective Support Systems

The first five modules of this manual dealt with the relationships between the care provider and the patient. Module VI deals with the patient care support systems that the care provider, whether family or professional, should cultivate and try to firmly establish. Care providers need to surround themselves with all of the components of an effective support system.

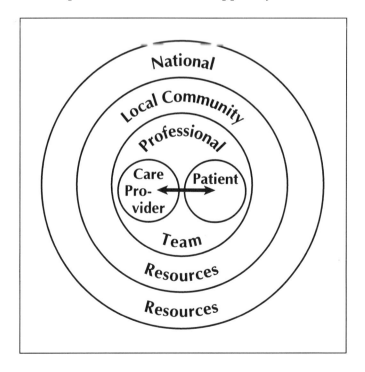

Suggested Resources on Aging, Dementia, and Related Subjects

The following agencies provide a variety of services, including referrals, general information, journals, and other types of publications:

Alzheimer's Disease and Related Disorders Association, 919 N. Michigan, Chicago, Illinois 60611-1616; phone 312 335-8700.

Alzheimer's Disease Education and Referral Center (ADEAR), P.O. Box 8250, Silver Spring, MD 20907; phone 301 495-3311

American Association of Homes for the Aging, Suite 400, 1129 20th Street, N.W., Washington, DC 20036; phone 202 783-2242

American Association of Retired Persons (AARP), 601 E Street, N.W., Washington, DC 20049; phone 202 434-2277

American Health Care Association, 1201 L Street, N.W., Washington, DC 20005; phone 202 842-4444

American Society on Aging, Suite 512, 833 Market Street, San Francisco, CA 94103; phone 415 974-9600

Assisted Living Facilities of America (ALFAA), 10300 Eaton Place, Suite 400, Fairfax, VA 22030; phone 703 691-8100

Family Caregiver Alliance, 425 Bush Street, Suite 500, San Francisco, CA 94108; phone 415 434-3388

Gerontological Society of America, 901 E Street, N.W., Suite 500, Washington, DC 20004; phone 202 842-1275

National Council on Aging, 409 3rd Street, S.W., Washington, DC 20024; phone 202 479-6998

National Hospice Organization, 1901 N. Moore Street, Suite 901, Arlington, VA 22209; phone 703 243-5900

National Institute on Aging, 315C 27 MSC 2292, 31 Center, Bethesda, MD 20892-2292; phone 301 496-1752

Helpful journals include:

American Journal of Alzheimer's Care and Related Disorders and Research, 470 Boston Post Road, Weston, MA 02193; phone 617 899-2702

Assisted Living Today: The Magazine of the Assisted Living Facilities Association of America, 10300 Eaton Place, Suite 400, Fairfax, VA 22030; phone 703 691-8100

Contemporary Long-Term Care Journal, 355 Park Avenue South, New York, NY 10010-1789; phone 212 592-6200

Geriatric Nursing, Mosby Yearbook, Inc., 1183 Westline Industrial Drive, St. Louis, MO 63146-3318; phone 314 872-8370

Nontraditional Family Units

Professional care providers need to know and understand the type of family structure of which the patient is a part. The traditional family units, in which an elderly dementia patient is cared for by a spouse of many years or by an adult child and the child's spouse, are no longer the only common types of family unit involved. Other fairly common types of family units, or units that are not even "family" in the traditional sense but that are providing care for a dementia patient, include:

a single adult child providing care, who may also have the sole care of
  young children;

a stepchild providing care for the spouse of a remarried father or mother;

a newly married spouse caring for a husband of only a few years (often
  with a shaky relationship with any stepchildren who may be involved);

an elderly sibling providing care for a brother or sister;

a remarried child caring for a parent along with stepchildren in the home;

nieces and nephews providing care;

same-sex couples providing care for one of the partner's parents, with or
  without children also in the home;

one of the partners in a same-sex relationship caring for the other with
  dementia;

a close friend providing care, with no involvement from any actual family
  members;

a traditional family in which there are several children, but who move the
  parent with dementia from home to home, sharing the care over a period
  of months or years;

grown grandchildren providing care for a grandparent.

Treating Others Objectively:

An Invaluable Skill

The following three principles necessary for successful, unbiased interaction with others have been adapted from the characteristics of a successful therapist as stated by psychologist Carl Rogers (see books by Rogers in the Bibliography). They are the basis for objective assessment of and positive interaction with dementia patients and their families.

1. Act genuinely interested in the other person. Try to get to know the person. Carl Rogers called this *congruence.* Be friendly and open; show interest; be alert. Listen to, observe, and think carefully about the person and what he or she is saying. Ask questions to draw the person out and learn more about him or her.

2. Put yourself in the person's situation. Think: "How would I feel if I were in his or her shoes?" Carl Rogers called this *empathy.* Think about the person's background and current status, then think how you would feel if you were in the same situation as this person with dementia or as this family member. Be careful not to identify too much, however. A professional should not get overly emotionally involved, or it becomes difficult to evaluate accurately and effectively.

3. Accept the person as he or she is without judgment, at all times, regardless of the person's behavior. Carl Rogers called this *unconditional positive regard.* Don't get angry, judge behavior, or try to argue. The dementia patient and the family need the support of a sympathetic listener who will not judge them. People with dementia act the way they do because of the disease. Accept the behavior the way you would the symptom of any disease. The family is going through an extremely difficult time, and your job is to help them get through it with the most positive outcome possible for them and for the patient.

Losses Families May Experience
When a Family Member Has Dementia

Loss of the person's companionship

Loss of someone to give emotional support

Loss of someone to talk with and confide in

Loss of free time

Loss of independence and ability to come and go freely

Lack of understanding from friends and relatives

Loss of emotional support or assistance from friends or relatives because they
    do not understand the need

Loss of the companionship of friends and relatives who may stop visiting or
    going out with the family because they do not understand

Diminished financial resources

Loss of hopes and dreams for the future

Fear of what the future may bring

Loss of sleep and adequate rest

Fear of loss or loss of their own health

Case Studies: Family Caregivers

Joe's Family

Joe was a high-functioning dementia patient with few behavior problems. He was a pleasure to have at the adult day care center and actively participated in all activities. He and his wife, May, had few close friends nearby. They had no children. Their relationship had never been very good, and May was constantly complaining about how difficult he was to care for. She never spoke about him in a positive way. They had little money, but she desperately looked for a residential care facility for him which she could afford, and finally placed him.

May's score on the burden interview was among the highest of all family members using the center at that time.

Sam's Family

Sam was a day care patient several years ago. He lived with his wife of sixty-five years, Ann. He had been diagnosed with dementia eight years earlier. He could no longer feed himself and was unaware of others at the center. He exhibited no real behavior problems but wandered the center and needed almost total care. His daughter, Suzanne, had her own family and was a schoolteacher. However, she brought him to the day center for her mother three days a week for a year. It then became too difficult for her to bring him each day because he had

H VI : 7

declined physically and could no longer walk or even transfer without a great deal of assistance.

At this point, Ann, who was eighty-five years old, continued to care for Sam at home. She had occasional help from Suzanne, who lived nearby and obviously loved and respected both of her parents very much. Ann and her daughter both continued to come to a support group at the center for awhile and frequently spoke of what a fine husband and father Sam had been and of the wonderful career as a music teacher he had achieved. Ann and Suzanne eventually stopped coming to the support group and lost touch with the center. However, after another year had gone by, Ann called the center one day to tell the staff Sam had died. It was obvious that she missed him very much and would continue to do so, probably until her own death.

While Sam attended the center, Ann had the lowest burden interview score of any family member using the center at that time.

Paul's Family

Susan and her husband, Michael, care for his father, Paul, a fairly young second-stage Alzheimer patient. They also have two young children. Even though Paul is declining, he has no severe behavior problems, and they have a large home with plenty of room for the whole family. Susan seems to be quite fond of Paul and has stated that they have always been close. However, Michael travels a lot, and she is left at home alone with Paul and the two children much of the time. Susan always talks to the social worker for a few minutes when she comes to pick up Paul at the adult day center, which he attends every day. She states frequently that it was Michael's idea to have Paul live with them and that he had promised to help with his father's care. She feels Paul is declining rapidly, even though he is still quite high functioning, and she usually mentions some new problem she is having with his care at home. She then asks if any new problems have been noted at the center.

QUESTIONS ABOUT THIS CASE STUDY:

Is there anything Susan is trying to say to the social worker beneath the actual verbal message? Does she just need to tell someone about the situation at home, or is there more involved?

Is the physical or the emotional burden of Paul's care probably greater for Susan?

What would your feelings be toward Susan? What would you say to her?

ACTUAL CONCLUSION OF THIS CASE STUDY:

There could be many answers to the above questions, but in this actual case, Susan finally admitted to the social worker that she really wanted to place Paul but felt very guilty about it and was afraid of what her husband would think. A few staff members expressed some anger toward Susan in staff meetings. They felt that she should be encouraged to try to accept the responsibility. In a conference with the social worker, Michael agreed to try to stay home more and provide more help. This worked for awhile, but as Paul grew worse, Michael also admitted that they could no longer care for him, especially with their young children to care for. They placed Paul soon after.

Organizational Chart

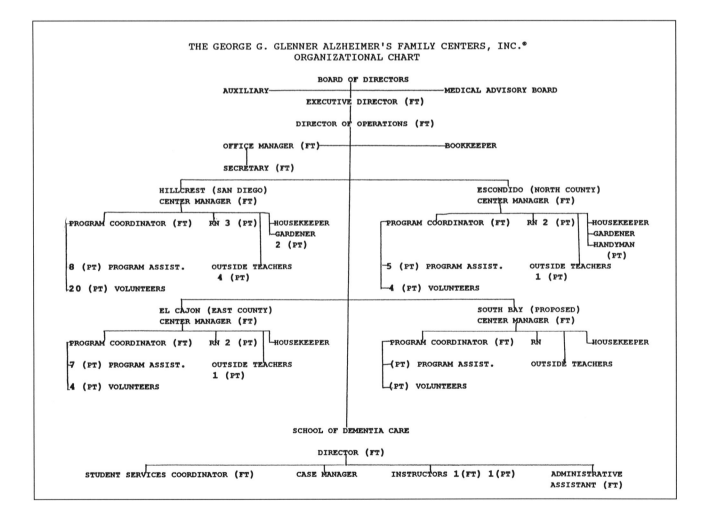

THE GEORGE G. GLENNER ALZHEIMER'S FAMILY CENTERS, INC.®
ORGANIZATIONAL CHART

BOARD OF DIRECTORS

AUXILIARY———————————————————————MEDICAL ADVISORY BOARD

EXECUTIVE DIRECTOR (FT)

DIRECTOR OF OPERATIONS (FT)

OFFICE MANAGER (FT)————————————————BOOKKEEPER

SECRETARY (FT)

HILLCREST (SAN DIEGO)
CENTER MANAGER (FT)

PROGRAM COORDINATOR (FT)   RN 3 (PT)   HOUSEKEEPER
                                         GARDENER
                                         2 (PT)

8 (PT) PROGRAM ASSIST.   OUTSIDE TEACHERS
                          4 (PT)
20 (PT) VOLUNTEERS

ESCONDIDO (NORTH COUNTY)
CENTER MANAGER (FT)

PROGRAM COORDINATOR (FT)   RN 2 (PT)   HOUSEKEEPER
                                         GARDENER
                                         HANDYMAN
                                         (PT)

5 (PT) PROGRAM ASSIST.   OUTSIDE TEACHERS
                          1 (PT)
4 (PT) VOLUNTEERS

EL CAJON (EAST COUNTY)
CENTER MANAGER (FT)

PROGRAM COORDINATOR (FT)   RN 2 (PT)   HOUSEKEEPER

7 (PT) PROGRAM ASSIST.   OUTSIDE TEACHERS
                          1 (PT)
4 (PT) VOLUNTEERS

SOUTH BAY (PROPOSED)
CENTER MANAGER (FT)

PROGRAM COORDINATOR (FT)   RN   HOUSEKEEPER

(PT) PROGRAM ASSIST.   OUTSIDE TEACHERS

(PT) VOLUNTEERS

SCHOOL OF DEMENTIA CARE

DIRECTOR (FT)

STUDENT SERVICES COORDINATOR (FT)   CASE MANAGER   INSTRUCTORS 1(FT) 1(PT)   ADMINISTRATIVE
                                                                                ASSISTANT (FT)

Job Description

Department: ADULT DAY CENTER
Position Title: PROGRAM ASSISTANT
Reports to: PROGRAM COORDINATOR

Qualifications:

1. Preference shall be given to certified nurse assistants, home health aides, and activity assistants or the equivalent. Must be bilingual—English and Spanish.
2. One year's work with the chronically impaired adult.
3. High school education or equivalent.
4. Able to communicate in English orally and in writing.
5. Physically able to perform the requirements of the position.
6. Able to properly interact with staff, patients, families, and volunteers.
7. Able to comply with state and county licensing regulations.
8. Able to comprehend and follow policies and procedures.

Position Summary: assist the activity coordinator with program activities for individual patients and groups of patients on a daily basis. Assist with each patient as needed with the program goals.

Salary Range: $12,000 to $18,000

Duties/Responsibilities:

1. Assist with:
   a. patient personal care and activities of daily living, such as toileting, feeding, walks, food preparation, etc.;
   b. observation and monitoring patient status during center hours and reporting same to supervisor;
   c. writing patient daily assessments;
   d. large and small group activities;
   e. planning and initiating appropriate parallel programing;
   f. one-to-one activities relating to each patient;
   g. setup and cleanup of activities.
2. Under the direction of a supervisor, plan and learn designated activities.
3. Occasionally may be requested to run errands, shop, or do light housekeeping.
4. Attend assigned staff meetings and in-service training sessions.
5. Report all emergencies to the supervisor.
6. Communicate within approved organizational structure.
7. Abide by policies and procedures.
8. Other duties as assigned.

This position is nonexempt from regulations of the Fair Labor Standards Act.

Employees with Pride in Their Profession:

The Basis for an Outstanding Agency or Facility

When a family visits an agency or facility they are considering for care of their family member with dementia, their concern is whether the agency will provide true caring of a consistently high quality. A good staff and pleasant surroundings make positive first impressions. Dedicated, caring staff members who present themselves in a *professional* manner are the best assets an agency can have. And remember, the maintenance of high personal standards not only is good for an agency but also helps ensure professional success as well! Important qualities for all professionals to develop and nurture are listed below.

Believe in the value of your profession

1. Know the profession. A thorough knowledge of the field is *essential.*
2. Know the specific job and what the agency stands for—the mission and goals of the agency.
3. Understand and believe in the value of your profession, your agency, and your specific job.
4. Consistently try to understand and *genuinely respect* all of your patients and their families.
5. Try not to be satisfied with "average"; continue to learn more about your profession and your job.

Maintain high standards of ethical conduct

1. Consistently perform your job as well as you possibly can.
2. Try to present your profession, your agency, and your specific job in a positive way at all times in public. Negative comments can be overheard and misconstrued on or off the job.
3. Never discuss patients or families outside the work place; confidentiality is essential in the caregiving professions.
4. Think before you speak. Learn to communicate and solve problems effectively with other members of your team.
5. Try to act calm and confident even when very stressed or angry. Smooth relationships between staff, families, and patients are essential to a smoothly running agency or facility. Discuss problems in private and when you are calm and can solve them constructively.
6. Conduct yourself in a manner that would be a credit to your profession and to your agency any time you are in public.
7. Unprofessional behavior, even far away from work, can come back to haunt you!

Take pride in your appearance

1. Dress appropriately for the job.
2. Maintain a neat appearance.
3. Maintain high standards of cleanliness.
4. Carry yourself with confidence. Posture and movements say a lot about you.
5. Remember that others get an impression of you from your office or work space. Maintain it in as orderly manner as your duties allow.

Stress Style Test: Body, Mind, or Mixed?

Imagine yourself in a stressful situation. When you're feeling anxious, what do you typically experience? (Check all that apply.)

___ 1. My heart beats faster.

___ 2. I find it difficult to concentrate because of distracting thoughts.

___ 3. I worry too much about things that don't really matter.

___ 4. I feel jittery.

___ 5. I get diarrhea.

___ 6. I imagine terrifying scenes.

___ 7. I can't keep anxiety-provoking pictures and images out of my mind.

___ 8. My stomach gets tense.

___ 9. I pace up and down nervously.

___ 10. I'm bothered by unimportant thoughts running through my mind.

___ 11. I become immobilized.

___ 12. I feel I'm losing out on things because I can't make decisions fast enough.

___ 13. I perspire.

___ 14. I can't stop thinking worrisome thoughts.

There are three basic ways of reacting to stress: primarily physical, mainly mental, or mixed. Physical stress types feel tension in the body—jitters, butterflies, the sweats. Mental types experience stress mainly in the mind—worries and preoccupying thoughts. Mixed types react with both responses in about equal measure.

Give yourself a Mind point if you answered "yes" to each of the following questions: 2, 3, 6, 7, 10, 12, 14. Give yourself a Body point for each of these: 1, 4, 5, 8, 9, 11, 13.

If you have more Mind than Body points, consider yourself a mental stress type. If you have more Body than Mind points, your stress style is physical. About the same number of each? You're a mixed reactor.

SOURCE: Daniel Goleman. 1986. "What's Your Stress Style?" *American Health Magazine,* April, p. 45. Reprinted with permission.

Choosing a Relaxer

Body: If stress registers mainly in your body, you'll need a remedy that will break up the physical tension pattern. This may be a vigorous body workout, but a slow-paced, even lazy, muscle relaxer may be equally effective. Here are some suggestions to get you started:

Aerobics	Walking
Swimming	Yoga
Body scan	Massage
Biking	Progressive relaxation
Rowing	Soaking in a hot tub, sauna

Mind: If you experience stress as an invasion of worrisome thoughts, the most direct intervention is anything that will engage your mind completely and redirect it—meditation, for example. On the other hand, some people find the sheer exertion of heavy physical exercise unhooks the mind wonderfully and is very fine therapy. Suggestions:

Knitting, sewing, carpentry, and other handicrafts	Games likes chess or cards
Meditation	Any absorbing hobby
Autogenic suggestion	Reading
Crossword puzzles	Vigorous exercise
	Television, movies

Mind/body: If you're a mixed type, you may want to try a physical activity that also demands mental rigor:

Competitive sports (racquetball, tennis, squash, volleyball, etc.)
Meditation

Any combination from the Mind and Body lists

SOURCE: Daniel Goleman. 1986. "What's Your Stress Style?" *American Health Magazine,* April, p. 45. Reprinted with permission.

The Body Scan

Here's a simplified version of the body scan. Once you've mastered it, you can scan anytime your body needs a quick tension review or you feel an overall need to calm down. During practice sessions, protect yourself from distractions and give yourself plenty of time to scan slowly and carefully. Wear comfortable clothes and lie on your back on a soft but firm surface. (After you learn the technique, you can do it in any position.) Spread your feet several inches apart, arms firmly at your sides. Now close your eyes and focus your attention on your breathing. Don't try to control your breathing—just become keenly aware of how it feels. Notice how your stomach and chest rise and fall with each breath. Or note the cool flow of air into your nose and the warm flow back out. Concentrate on whatever sensations interest you.

Here's the basic technique: Each time you inhale, scan a muscle area. As you exhale, try to release the tension there. As you become aware of tension in a muscle zone, imagine each out-breath draining it away. Stay in each region for a long, still moment. Breathe in, breathe out. Linger wherever it's needed. Don't worry if your mind wanders while you're scanning. Just bring your attention back to the last point in the scan and continue. First, bring your awareness to your head and face. Tour your whole head with your mind's eye—your scalp, the back and sides of your head, forehead and temples, eyes and nose, cheeks and mouth, jaws and chin. Take plenty of time. Observe any sensations you find there as you inhale, and imagine the tension melting away as you exhale. On every in-breath, scan; on every out-breath, release. Feel the tension slipping away as you exhale.

Using this technique, move down through your body, focusing next on your neck, shoulders, and arms. Then go on to chest and stomach, back, and, finally, legs and feet. Breathe in, breathe out. Don't rush—there's lots to notice in each area. Whenever you feel tension, scan the in-breath, release on the out. Feel a deepening relaxation as you move through your tension spots, relaxing the tightness, leaving the muscle soft, heavy, and warm.

When you've finished, lie there limp. Notice what it's like to be completely relaxed, yet alert and aware. Take a few deep breaths and get up slowly. Keep this feeling of relaxation as you return to your daily activities.

There's always another scan.

SOURCE: Daniel Goleman. 1986. "What's Your Stress Style?" *American Health Magazine,* April, p. 44. Reprinted with permission.

Glossary

Active aging The healthier lifestyle of older adults who make a conscious effort to keep physically, mentally, and socially active.

Activities of Daily Living (ADLs) The basic personal care tasks that must be performed to maintain some degree of independence, such as eating, transferring, walking inside and out, dressing, grooming, bathing, and toileting.

Acute condition A disease or symptom that appears very suddenly with marked intensity and subsides in a relatively short period of time.

Addison disease A disease due to deficient functioning of the adrenal glands, causing severe weakness, diarrhea, loss of weight, low blood pressure, and dementia. The condition is usually fatal within two to three years.

Agnosia The loss of the ability to recognize familiar objects by sight, touch, taste, smell, or sound.

Alzheimer disease A disease with the primary symptom of progressive dementia; characterized by progressive, irreversible, and lethal structural damage to the brain due to the presence of abnormal proteins.

Aphasia The inability to form words or express oneself clearly orally or in writing is *expressive aphasia*. The inability or decreased ability to understand spoken or written language is *receptive aphasia*.

Apraxia The loss of the ability to carry out complex learned motor movements.

Assessment An evaluation of a condition. Careful and complete initial and ongoing assessment is vital to therapeutic care of dementia patients.

Autopsy A postmortem examination performed to determine the cause of death.

Behavior problem Any type of problem which is harmful, potentially harmful, or disturbing to the person performing the action or to others. Such problems are very common among dementia patients due to damage to the brain caused by the disease process.

Benign forgetfulness (or *benign senescence*) The slowing of some mental powers normal in aging. It is not dementia, and dementia is not normal aging.

Brain bank A depository of brain tissue for use in diagnosing disease and to supply human tissue for research.

Caregiver A person responsible for most or all of the care of another human being.

Care plan A document specifying long-term care goals for patients and the time frame within which the goals are to be reached. Goals are determined through careful assessment of the patient's physical and psychosocial problems. These problems, approaches, and goals should be identified by the entire professional team involved.

Catastrophic reaction A fairly sudden negative change in the behavior of a dementia patient which can occur for a wide variety of reasons.

Chronic condition A disease or disorder that develops slowly and persists over a long period of time.

Cognition All the components of the mental process. These include awareness and comprehension of ideas, things, and events; retention of the experience; retrieval of it; sequencing ideas, forming concepts, and learning from them; reasoning and forming judgments and opinions.

Delusion A persistent belief that an event or situation is true even though it may be illogical. It is often based on fact or a distortion of facts.

Dementia A global, long-lasting decline in intellectual functioning caused by disease or other injury to the brain.

Depression An abnormal emotional state characterized by feelings of worthlessness, sadness, emptiness, and hopelessness. When the primary diagnosis of the mental disorder is depression, it is potentially reversible but is often extremely difficult to treat. It may be so severe that physical symptoms and symptoms of mental impairment (including short- and long-term memory loss, confusion, delusions, and hallucinations) occur. When the symptoms of dementia appear but do not have an organic base, it is a *pseudodementia*. Depression is the most common pseudodementia. Alzheimer and related diseases, therapeutic drug use, and illegal drug use can all cause depression as a symptom of the primary condition.

Diagnosis The identification of a disease or condition by scientific examination of physical signs and symptoms, history, laboratory tests, and other procedures.

Excess disability The disability that a patient displays beyond what should be present as a result of the true level of impairment.

Fine-motor functions Small, controlled movements of the muscles of the body. A good example is the controlled movement of the fingers, wrist, hand, and arm in order to paint or draw.

Functional disability The inability of a person to perform one or more of the ADLs/IADLs, resulting in the need for total help from another person in the affected areas.

Functional limitation The reduced ability of a person to perform one or more of the ADLs/IADLs; some assistance from a device or community service, but not the constant assistance of another person, is needed to perform the tasks affected.

Gene The basic unit of genetic material (composed of specific nucleic acids) determining each living organism's biological composition based on heredity.

Genetic Produced by a gene; inherited.

Hallucination A persistent belief that something is seen, heard, or smelled, when nothing is really there. It is not based on fact, or even misinterpretation of fact.

History A document recording all relevant medical *(the medical history)* or psychosocial *(the social history)* information about a patient or resident to enable the caregiver to care for the person to the best of his or her ability.

Huntington disease A rare, abnormal hereditary condition characterized by involuntary, purposeless movements and progressive dementia. Patients usually begin to have symptoms in their forties and have a life expectancy of approximately fifteen more years.

Incontinence The loss of bowel and bladder control due to physical problems or to an inability to perceive signals correctly, which is common in Alzheimer disease.

Instrumental Activities of Daily Living (IADLs) The tasks of home management (such as money management, shopping, housekeeping, preparing meals, and answering the telephone) that are necessary but not as crucial to independent living as the ADLs.

Irreversible dementia A type of dementia which can never be treated and alleviated but which may be *nonprogressive:* it may not become worse with time. A *progressive* irreversible dementia will get worse and is ultimately *lethal:* it will cause death. Dementia of the Alzheimer type is the most common irreversible, progressive, lethal dementia.

Korsakoff syndrome A condition often seen in chronic alcoholism and caused by degenerative changes in the brain. It is characterized in part by short-term memory loss and an inability to learn new skills.

Language Words, their pronunciation, and the combinations that people use to express themselves. The understanding and retention of spoken or written language is *receptive language.* The ability to communicate orally or in writing is *expressive language.* Speech is the ability to enunciate expressive language correctly.

Large-motor functions Wide, expansive movements of the large muscles of the body. Swinging a leg or an arm is an example of large-motor movement.

Level of care The amount of physical care, psychosocial stimulation, and supervision a resident or patient requires; measured by the staff-to-patient ratio, kind of staff, and type of care needed to provide good-quality care for that person.

Metabolic disorder Dysfunction of the chemical balance in the body, which must be maintained to properly control growth, generation of energy, elimination of waste, etc.

Multi-infarct dementia A dementia caused by small cerebrovascular accidents that may be so small that the individual accidents can go undetected, but which eventually result in a stepwise deterioration of cognitive functioning.

Neurology The field of medicine dealing with the nervous system; composed of the brain, spinal cord, and cranial and spinal nerves.

Parallel programing The provision of two or more simultaneous activities for groups or individuals, each designed to meet the differing needs of the specific individuals or groups.

Parkinson disease A slowly progressive neurological disorder usually occurring in the early sixties, characterized by tremor, masklike facial features, rolling gait, and other muscular disturbances. Symptoms of dementia can occur, or occur as a result of medication for other symptoms of the disease.

Passive aging A decline in physical and/or emotional health and/or social involvement of older people caused by their inability or lack of desire to adapt to the physical and emotional changes associated with normal aging.

Pathology The study of the characteristics, causes, and effects of disease by examining the structural and functional changes in the body.

Perception The conscious recognition and interpretation of external stimuli using any of the senses. Correct interpretation is based on unconscious association with memory and is the basis for correct understanding and learning of new information.

Perseveration The compulsive repetition of a simple one- or two-step action over and over again. It is characteristic of patients with a dementia. Once the patient has grasped the ability to perform a simple action, it is often done repeatedly and is difficult to stop. If the perseveration is not harmful in any way, it can be beneficial, since the patient has the satisfaction of performing an activity independently, something dementia patients can seldom accomplish.

Pick disease A disease affecting the frontal and temporal lobes of the brain and causing early dementia, usually in middle age.

Positive interaction techniques The specific types of communicative techniques essential for use with dementia patients to maintain a positive, productive emotional climate and working relationship.

Psychiatric disorder Any disturbance of emotional, behavioral, or functional ability caused by genetic, physical, chemical, social, or cultural factors.

Psychosocial Having to do with a person's mental health, social status, and ability to function in the community.

Psychotropic drugs Those drugs primarily designed to affect the brain, controlling emotions and behavior. Psychotropic drugs are not only tranquilizers; some act as antidepressants, others can reduce anxiety.

Sundowner syndrome Confusion and irritation common in dementia patients at the end of the day. The cause of Sundowner syndrome is not really known, but it may be due to general tiredness and an inability to process any more information or to interpret the environment correctly. A reduced level of activity consisting of familiar, undemanding tasks is best at this time.

Therapeutic activity Any activity that a person enjoys and that has positive meaning for the person. A *therapeutic program* is a total program of care based on a complete assessment and specifically designed to meet these needs and keep the person functioning at the highest possible level in all areas.

Bibliography

Abrams, William; Berkow, Robert; and Fletcher, Andrew J. 1990. *The Merck Manual of Geriatrics.* Rahway, N.J.: Merck Sharp and Dohme Research Laboratories.

Abrass, Itamar B.; Kane, Robert L.; and Ouslander, Joseph G. 1989. *Essentials of Clinical Geriatrics,* 2d ed. New York: McGraw-Hill.

Adams, Hume; Corsellis, J.A.N; and Duchen, L. W., eds. 1984. *Greenfield's Neuropathology.* New York: Wiley.

Alzheimer's Disease and Related Disorders Association. 1992. *Dental Care Action Steps.* Chicago: Alzheimer's Disease and Related Disorders Association.

———. 1992. *Guidelines for Dignity: Goals of Specialized Alzheimer/Dementia Care in Residential Settings.* Chicago: Alzheimer's Disease and Related Disorders Association.

Andrews, Jane. 1989. *Poverty and Poor Health among Elderly Hispanic Americans.* Baltimore: Commonwealth Fund Commission.

Baggett, Sharon A., and Pratt, Clara. 1992. *An Oregon Guide to Special Care Units for Persons with Dementia.* Corvallis: Oregon State University.

Ballard, Edna L., and Poer, Cornelia M. 1992. *Sexuality and the Alzheimer's Patient.* Durham, N.C.: Duke Family Support Program, Duke University Medical Center.

Barinaga, Marcia. 1993. Neuroscientists Reach a Critical Mass in Washington. *Science* 262:1210–11.

Bartol, Mari Ann. 1979. Nonverbal Communication in Patients with Alzheimer's Disease. *Journal of Gerontology* 5:21–32, July.

Baugh, Mary Francis. 1991. *When a Loved One Has Alzheimer's.* St. Meinrad, Ind.: Abbey Press.

Berkow, Robert, and Fletcher, Andrew J., eds. 1987. *The Merck Manual of Diagnosis and Therapy.* Rahway, N.J.: Merck Sharp and Dohme Research Laboratories.

Boccia, Aldo. 1992. Alzheimer's Disease and the Dental Patient. *Ontario Dentist,* 16–18:Apr.

Bosshardt, John P.; Gibson, Dorothy E.; and Snyder, Marolyn. 1979. *Family Survival Handbook: A Guide to the Financial, Legal, and Social Problems of Brain Damaged Adults.* San Francisco: Family Survival Project.

Boyd, Rosangela K.; James, Anne; and McGuire, Francis. 1992. *Therapeutic Humor with the Elderly.* Binghamton, N.Y.: Haworth Press.

Brammer, Lawrence M. 1991. *How to Cope with Life Transitions: The Challenge of Personal Change.* New York: Hemisphere.

Brawley, Elizabeth. 1992. Alzheimer's Disease: Designing the Physical Environment. *American Journal of Alzheimer's Care and Related Disorders and Research,* 11K–11P:Jan./Feb.

Brechling, Brigid G.; Heyworth, Judith A.; Kuhn, Dan; and Peranteau, Mary F. 1989. Extending Hospice Care to End-Stage Dementia Patients and Families. *American Journal of Alzheimer's Care and Related Disorders and Research,* 21–29:May/June.

Brink, T. L. 1986. *Clinical Gerontology: A Guide to Assessment and Intervention.* New York: Haworth Press.

Brody, Elaine M.; Lawton, Powell M.; and Saperstein, Avalia R. 1991. *Respite for Caregivers of Alzheimer Patients: Research and Practice.* New York: Springer.

Brown, Stephen. 1988. *When Your Rope Breaks.* Nashville: Thomas Nelson.

Buckman, Robert. 1992. *How to Break Bad News: A Guide for Health Care Professionals.* Baltimore: Johns Hopkins University Press.

Buys, Donna, and Saltman, Jules. 1982. *The Elderly, the Unseen Alcoholics.* New York: Public Affairs Committee.

Cacioppo, Paul P. 1992. *Health Care Fraud and Abuse: A Guide to Federal Sanctions.* New York: Clark Boardman Callaghan.

Carey, Joseph. 1992. *How the Brain Ages.* Washington, D.C.: Society for Neuroscience.

Caron, Wayne. 1992. *A Family Systems Model for Dementia of the Alzheimer's Type.* Minneapolis: University of Minnesota, Department of Family Practice and Community Health.

Caruana, Claudia M. 1985. How to Overcome Stress. *Consumers Digest,* 30–34:Oct.

Charlesworth, Edward A., and Nathan, Ronald G. 1984. *Stress Management: A Comprehensive Guide to Wellness.* New York: Atheneum.

Clark, Cheryl. 1994. If This Is the Cause, Cure Could Be Next. *San Diego Union-Tribune,* E-1, E-4, Sept.

Cleland, Marilyn, and Schmall, Vicki L. 1990. *Helping Memory-Impaired Elders: A Guide for Caregivers.* Portland: Pacific Northwest Extension Service.

Cluff, Pamela J. 1990. Alzheimer's Disease and the Institution: Issues in Environmental Design. *American Journal of Alzheimer's Care and Related Disorders and Research,* 23–32:May/June.

Cohen, Donna. 1991. The Subjective Experience of Alzheimer's Disease: The Anatomy of an Illness as Perceived by Patients and Families. *American Journal of Alzheimer's Care and Related Disorders and Research,* 6–11:May/June.

Cohen, Donna, and Eisdorfer, Carl. 1986. *The Loss of Self: A Family Resource for the Care of Alzheimer's Disease and Related Disorders.* New York: New American Library.

Cohen, Pat Stacey, and Sincox, Rochelle. 1986. *Adapting the Adult Day Care Environment for Older Adults with Dementia.* Winnetka: Illinois Department of Aging.

Cohen, Uriel, and Day, Kristen. 1993. *Contemporary Environments for People with Dementia.* Baltimore: Johns Hopkins University Press.

Cohen, Uriel, and Weisman, Gerald D. 1991. *Holding On to Home: Designing Environments for People with Dementia.* Baltimore: Johns Hopkins University Press.

Cole, Thomas; Van Tassel, David D.; and Kastenbaum, Robert. 1992. *Handbook of the Humanities and Aging.* New York: Springer.

Coons, Dorothy H. 1988. Wandering. *American Journal of Alzheimer's Care and Related Disorders and Research*, 31–36:Jan./Feb.

———, ed. 1990. *Specialized Dementia Care Units*. Baltimore: Johns Hopkins University Press.

Coons, Dorothy H., and Reichel, William. 1988. Improving the Quality of Life in Nursing Homes. *American Family Physicians* 37:241–48.

Coons, Dorothy; Metzelaar, Lena; Robinson, Anne; and Spencer, Beth. 1986. *A Better Life: Helping Family Members, Volunteers, and Staff Improve the Quality of Life of Nursing Home Residents Suffering from Alzheimer's Disease and Related Disorders*. Columbus, Ohio: Source for Nursing Home Literature.

Coughlan, Patricia Brown. 1993. *Facing Alzheimer's: Family Caregivers Speak*. New York: Ballantine Books.

Crabtree, Jill, and Quinn, Terry. 1987. *How to Take Care of You—So You Can Take Care of Others*. Downers Grove, Ill.: Heritage Arts.

Cronk, Renee. 1993. *Fact Sheet: Selected Caregiver Statistics*. San Francisco: Family Caregiver Alliance.

Cunninghis, Richelle N. 1990. *Quality Assurance for Activity Programs: A How-To Manual*. Willingboro, N.J.: Geriatric Educational Consultants.

Curran, Charles E. 1978. *Issues in Sexual and Medical Ethics*. Notre Dame, Ind.: University of Notre Dame Press.

Davis, Martha; Eshelman, E. R.; and McKay, Matthew. 1982. *The Relaxation and Stress Reduction Workbook*. Oakland: New Harbinger.

Dawson, Pam; Kline, Karen; Wiancko, Donna Crinklaw; and Wells, Donna. 1986. Preventing Excess Disability in Patients with Alzheimer's Disease. *Geriatric Nursing*, 298–301:Nov./Dec.

Dickman, Irving R. 1981. *Listen to Your Body: Exercise and Physical Fitness*. New York: Public Affairs Committee.

———. 1988. *Macular Degeneration: Vision Impairment of the Later Years*. New York: Public Affairs Committee.

Donius, Maggie, and Rader, Joanne. 1991. *Magic, Mystery, Modification, and Mirth: The Joyful Road to Restraint-Free Care*. Mt. Angel, Ore.: Benedictine Institute for Long Term Care.

Doukas, David John, and Reichel, William. 1993. *Planning for Uncertainty: A Guide to Living Wills and Other Advance Directives for Health Care*. Baltimore: Johns Hopkins University Press.

Dowling, James R. 1995. *Keeping Busy: A Handbook of Activities for Persons with Dementia*. Baltimore: Johns Hopkins University Press.

Down, Ivy, and Schnurr, Lorraine. 1991. *Between Home and Nursing Home: The Board and Care Alternative*. Buffalo: Prometheus Books.

Duffy, Linda M. 1993. *The Tie That Binds: An Exploration in Sexual Intimacy of Alzheimer's Couples*. Minneapolis: Geriatric Research, Education, and Clinical Center, Minneapolis V.A. Medical Center.

Eccles, Margaret. 1991. *Thesaurus of Aging Terminology*, 4th ed. Washington, D.C.: American Association of Retired Persons.

Edwards, Allen Jack. 1993. *Dementia*. New York: Plenum Press.

Enck, Robert E. 1992. Alzheimer's Disease. *American Journal of Hospice and Palliative Care*, 12–13:Sept./Oct.

Family Caregiver Alliance. 1993. *Community Care Options Fact Sheet*. San Francisco: Family Caregiver Alliance, June.

Fisher, Jeffrey A. 1992. *Rx 2000: Breakthroughs in Health, Medicine, and Longevity by the Year 2000 and Beyond*. New York: Simon and Schuster.

Flint, Alastair J. 1991. Delusions, Hallucinations, and Depression in Alzheimer's Disease: A Biological Perspective. *American Journal of Alzheimer's Care and Related Disorders and Research,* 21–28:May/June.

Freed, David M. 1984. Methods of Establishing a Clinical Diagnosis of Alzheimer's Disease. Ph.D. diss., Texas Tech University Health Sciences Center, Lubbock.

Freese, Arthur S. 1979. *Stroke: New Approaches to Prevention and Treatment.* New York: Public Affairs Committee.

———. 1981. *The Brain and Aging: The Myths, the Facts.* New York: Public Affairs Committee.

French, Carolyn; Levine, Eve; and Morrison, Nancy. 1990. *Guide to Home Safety for Caregivers of Persons with Alzheimer's Disease.* Atlanta: Atlanta Area Chapter, Alzheimer's Association.

Friedan, Betty. 1993. *The Fountain of Age.* New York: Simon and Schuster.

Gaberlavage, George; Moon, Marilyn; and Newman, Sandra J. 1985. *Preserving Independence, Supporting Needs: The Role of Board and Care Homes.* Washington, D.C.: Public Policy Institute, American Association of Retired Persons.

Gates, Philomene. 1990. *Suddenly Alone: A Woman's Guide to Widowhood.* New York: Harper Perennial.

Gilford, Dorothy M. 1988. *The Aging Population in the Twenty-first Century: Statistics for Health Policy.* Washington, D.C.: National Academy Press.

Gilster, Susan D., and McCracken, Ann L. 1989. Helping Alzheimer's Disease Caregivers Re-Establish Their Own Lives. *American Journal of Alzheimer's Care and Related Disorders and Research,* 14–18:Mar./Apr.

Glenner, George G. 1984. The Amyloid Deposits in Alzheimer's Disease: Their Nature and Pathogenesis. *Applied Pathology* 2:357–64.

———. 1988. Alzheimer's Disease: Its Proteins and Genes. *Cell* 52:307–8.

———. 1988. The Proteins and Genes of Alzheimer's Disease. *Biomedicine and Pharmacotherapy* 42:579–84.

———. 1992. Editorial: Converging Pathways in Alzheimer's Disease. *Laboratory Investigation* 67:271–73.

———. 1994. Alzheimer's Disease. In *Encyclopedia of Human Biology,* 1:103–11. New York: Academic Press.

Glenner, George G., and Wong, C. W. 1984. Alzheimer's Disease: Initial Report of the Purification and Characterization of a Novel Cerebrovascular Amyloid Protein. *Biochemical and Biophysical Research Communications* 120:885–90.

———. 1984. Alzheimer's Disease and Down's Syndrome: Sharing of a Unique Cerebrovascular Amyloid Fibril Protein. *Biochemical and Biophysical Research Communications* 122:1131–35.

Glenner, George G.; de Freitas, Falcao; and Pinho e Costa, Pedro. 1980. *Amyloid and Amyloidosis.* New York: Excerpta Medica.

Glenner, George G.; Quaranta, W. V.; and Wong, C. W. 1985. Neuritic Plaques and Cerebrovascular Amyloid in Alzheimer's Disease Are Antigenically Related. *Proceedings of the National Academy of Sciences, USA* 82:8729–32.

Glenner, Joy; Joiner, Judy; LeDuc, Janet; Neubauer, Judi; Stehman, Jean Mason; and Strachan, Geraldine. 1990. Alzheimer's Disease: A Study of Assessment and Stages. *American Journal of Alzheimer's Care and Related Disorders and Research* 5:28–36.

Glick, Ira O.; Weiss, Robert; and Parkes, Murray C. 1974. *The First Year of Bereavement.* New York: Wiley.

Goleman, Daniel. 1986. What's Your Stress Style? *American Health,* 44–45, Apr.

Goodrich, Theresa; Hedrick, Hannah L.; Isenberg, Daryl H.; Katz, Alfred H.; Kutscher, Austin H.; and Thompson, Leslie M. 1992. *Self-Help Concepts and Applications*. Philadelphia: Charles Press.

Gorden, Alex, and Saltman, Jules. 1979. *Know Your Medication: How to Use Over-the-Counter and Prescription Drugs*. New York: Public Affairs Committee.

Gray, David Dodson. 1993. *I Want to Remember: A Son's Reflection on His Mother's Alzheimer Journey*. Wellesley, Mass.: Roundtable Press.

Grollman, Earl A. 1980. *When Your Loved One Is Dying*. Boston: Beacon Press.

Gruetzner, Howard. 1988. *Alzheimer's: A Caregivers Guide and Source Book*. New York: Wiley.

Gugel, R. Nacken. 1988. Managing the Problematic Behaviors of the Alzheimer's Victim. *American Journal of Alzheimer's Care and Related Disorders and Research*, 12–15:May/June.

Gwyther, Lisa P. 1985. *Care of Alzheimer's Patients: A Manual for Nursing Home Staff*. Durham, N.C.: American Health Care Association and Alzheimer's Disease and Related Disorders Association.

Hawes, Catherine; Lux, Linda J.; and Wildfire, Judith B. 1993. *The Regulations of Board and Care Homes*. Washington, D.C.: American Association of Retired Persons.

Hirst, Sandra T., and Metcalf, Barbara J. 1989. Whys and Whats of Wandering. *Geriatric Nursing*, 237–38:Sept./Oct.

Hoffman, Stephanie, and Platt, Constance A. 1981. *Comforting the Confused: Strategies for Managing Dementia*. New York: Springer.

Honel, Rosalie Walsh. 1988. *Journey with Grandpa: Our Family's Struggle with Alzheimer's Disease*. Baltimore: Johns Hopkins University Press.

Hurley, Ann C.; Volicer, Beverly; Hanrahan, Patricia A.; Houde, Susan; and Volicer, Ladislav. 1992. Assessment of Discomfort in Advanced Alzheimer Patients. *Research in Nursing and Health*, 375-1–375-9.

Institute for Technology Development. 1991. *Design for Alzheimer's: A Bibliography*. Oxford, Miss.: Institute for Technology Development.

Irwin, Theodore. 1978. *Home Health Care: When a Patient Leaves the Hospital*. New York: Public Affairs Committee.

Jackson, J. E. 1992. Practical Pharmacology for the Elderly Patient in the Emergency Department. *Topics in Emergency Medicine* 14:10–19, Sept.

Jackson, J. E., and Ramsdell, J. W. 1989. *New Perspectives in Geriatric Medicine: Chronic Obstructive Pulmonary Disease*. Research Triangle Park, N.C.: Allen and Hanbury Division, Glaxo.

———. 1989. *New Perspectives in Geriatric Medicine: Cognitive Impairment*. Research Triangle Park, N.C.: Allen and Hanbury Division, Glaxo.

———. 1989. *New Perspectives in Geriatric Medicine: Gait Disorders*. Research Triangle Park, N.C.: Allen and Hanbury Division, Glaxo.

———. 1989. *New Perspectives in Geriatric Medicine: Hypertension*. Research Triangle Park, N.C.: Allen and Hanbury Division, Glaxo.

Jacob Perlow Hospice, Inc. 1989. *Possible Prognosticators of Death for Terminally Ill Patients with Alzheimer's Disease*. New York: Beth Israel Medical Center.

Janz, Marcie. 1990. Clues to Elder Abuse. *Geriatric Nursing*, 220–22:Sept./Oct.

Jarvik, Lissy, and Small, Gary. 1988. *Parent Care: A Common Sense Guide for Adult Children*. New York: Crown.

Jarvik, Lissy F.; Besdine, Richard W.; and Tangalos, Eric G. 1991. Managing Advanced Alzheimer's Disease. *Patient Care*, 75–100:Nov.

Jacobs, Geraldine. 1989. *Involving Men in Caregiver Support Groups: A Practical Guidebook*. Graduate School of Social Work and Social Research, Bryn Mawr College, Bryn Mawr, Pa.

Kievman, Beverly, and Blackman, Susie. 1989. *For Better or for Worse: A Couple's Guide to Dealing with Chronic Illness*. Chicago: Contemporary Books.

Kubler-Ross, Elizabeth. 1969. *On Death and Dying: What the Dying Have to Teach Doctors, Nurses, Clergy, and Their Own Families*. New York: Macmillan.

———. 1975. *Death: The Final Stage of Growth*. Englewood Cliffs, N.J.: Prentice-Hall.

Kushner, Harold S. 1983. *When Bad Things Happen to Good People*. New York: Avon Books.

Light, Enid, and Lebowitz, Barry D. 1990. *Alzheimer's Disease Treatment and Family Stress: Direction for Research*. New York: Hemisphere.

Lindeman, David; Corby, Nancy H.; Downing, Rachel; and Sanborn, Beverly. 1991. *Alzheimer's Day Care: A Basic Guide*. New York: Hemisphere.

Lyman, Karen A. 1993. *Day In, Day Out with Alzheimer's: Stress in Caregiving Relationships*. Philadelphia: Temple University Press.

McCabe, Barbara W.; Sand, Barbara J.; and Yeaworth, Rosalee C. 1992. Alzheimer's Disease Special Care Units in Long-Term Care Facilities. *Journal of Gerontological Nursing*, 28–34:Mar.

McDowell, Paul V., and Moore, Julie L. 1993. *Abstracts in Social Gerontology: Current Literature on Aging*. Washington, D.C.: Periodicals Press.

Mace, Nancy, ed. 1989. *Dementia Care: Patient, Family, and Community*. Baltimore: Johns Hopkins University Press.

Mace, Nancy, and Gwyther, Lisa P. 1989. *Selecting a Nursing Home with a Dedicated Dementia Care Unit*. Chicago: Alzheimer's Disease and Related Disorders Association.

Mace, Nancy, and Rabins, Peter V. 1991. *The 36-Hour Day: A Family Guide to Caring for Persons with Alzheimer's Disease, Related Dementing Illnesses, and Memory Loss in Later Life*, rev. ed. Baltimore: Johns Hopkins University Press.

Maddux, Robert B. 1988. *Team Building, an Exercise in Leadership: A Proven Way to Increase Organizational Effectiveness*. Los Altos, Calif.: Crisp Publications.

Manning, Doug. 1983. *When Love Gets Tough: The Nursing Home Decision*. Hereford, Tex.: Insight Books.

Markus, Karen. 1991. Durable Power of Attorney for Health Care. *California Nursing*, 20–24:July / Aug.

Marx, Jean. 1992. Boring in on B-Amyloid's Role in Alzheimer's. *Science* 255:688–89.

Miner, Gary D.; Winters-Miner, Linda A.; Blass, John P.; Richter, Ralph W.; and Valentine, Jimmie L. 1989. *Caring for Alzheimer's Patients: A Guide for Family and Health Care Providers*. New York: Plenum Press.

Moody, Harry R. 1992. *Ethics in an Aging Society*. Baltimore: Johns Hopkins University Press.

Morshita, Lynne; Sebastian-Moyer, Martha; Shultz, Judith; Specht, Claire; and Wilber, Kate. 1990. Working with the Difficult Elderly Client. *American Society on Aging*, May.

Murphey, Cecil. 1988. *Day to Day: Spiritual Help When Someone You Love Has Alzheimer's*. Philadelphia: Westminster Press.

Murphy, Mary Brugger. 1993. *A Manual for Training the Program Assistant in Adult Day Care*. Washington, D.C.: National Council on Aging.

Namazi, Kevin H. 1994. Research Brief: Attention Span. *Respite Report* 6:Winter.

Nissenboim, Sylvia, and Vroman, Christine. 1988. *Interactions by Design: The Positive Interactions Program for Persons with Alzheimer's Disease and Related Disorders*. St. Louis: Geri-Active Consultants.

Oates, Wayne. 1988. *Easing the Burden of Stress*. St. Meinrad, Ind.: Abbey Press.

Obade, Claire C. 1992. *Patient Care Decision Making: A Legal Guide for Providers*. Pub. no. 100-612. New York: Thomas Legal Publishing.

Ogg, Elizabeth. 1980. *The Right to Die with Dignity.* New York: Public Affairs Committee.

Olsen, Richard V.; Ehrenkrantz, Ezra; and Hutchings, Barbara M. 1993. *Homes That Help: Advice from Caregivers for Creating a Supportive Home.* Newark: NJIT Press.

Orr, Nancy; Zarit, Judy; and Zarit, Steven. 1985. *The Hidden Victims of Alzheimer's Disease: Families under Stress.* New York: New York University Press.

Peck, Carol. 1989. *Activities, Adaptations, and Aging from Deep Within: Poetry Workshop in Nursing Homes.* Vol. 13, no. 3. Binghamton, N.Y.: Haworth Press.

Peppard, Nancy R. 1991. *Special Needs Dementia Units: Design, Development, and Operations.* New York: Springer.

Peterson, James. 1988. Revised by Pamela Warrick. *On Being Alone: A Guide for Widowed Persons.* Washington, D.C.: American Association of Retired Persons.

Physicians Desk Reference, 49th ed. 1995. Montvale, N.J.: Medical Economics Data.

Podlosky, Doug, and Silberner, Joanne. 1993. How Medicine Mistreats the Elderly. *U.S. News and World Report,* 72–79, Jan. 18.

Pollen, Daniel A. 1993. *Hannah's Heirs: The Quest for the Genetic Origins of Alzheimer's Disease.* New York: Oxford University Press.

Posey Company. 1993. *The Posey Company Policy on the Use of Restraints.* Arcadia, Calif.: Posey Co.

Prather, Steve. 1992. Men's Activity Group for Early Diagnosed Alzheimer's Patients and Their Families. Ph.D. diss., Department of Psychobiology, University of California, Irvine, Research Unit in Brain Aging, Costa Mesa.

Pynoos, Jon, and Cohen, Evelyn. 1988. *Creating a Supportive Environment in Adult Day Care Centers: A Training Module and Slide Show.* Sacramento: California Department of Aging.

Rabins, Peter; Low, Randy; Morril, Elizabeth; Johnson, Lillian; and Smith, Sally. 1990. Perspectives on a Special Care Unit. *American Journal of Alzheimer's Care and Related Disorders and Research,* 13–21:Sept./Oct.

Rae, Stephen. 1994. Bright Light, Big Therapy. *MM,* 36–85:Feb./Mar.

Reif, Laura; Bould, Sally; and Sanborn, Beverly. 1989. *The Oldest Old: Eighty-Five Plus.* Belmont, Calif.: Wadsworth.

Riley, James F. 1988. Nursing Homes for Alzheimer's Patients Require Special Design. *Consulting Specifying Engineer,* 48–49:Aug.

Rofes, Eric E. 1985. The Unit at Fayerweather Street School. In *The Kid's Book about Death and Dying by the Kids.* Boston: Little, Brown.

Rogers, Carl R. 1961. *On Becoming a Person: A Therapist's View of Psychotherapy.* Boston: Houghton Mifflin.

Rogers, Carl R., and Stevens, Barry. 1967. *Person to Person: The Problem of Being Human.* Menlo Park, Calif.: Peninsula Lithograph.

Rovner, Barry W.; Broadhead, Jeremy; Spencer, Miriam; Carson, Kathryn; and Folstein, Marshall F. 1989. Depression and Alzheimer's Disease. *American Journal of Psychiatry* 146:350–52, Mar.

Sacks, Oliver. 1987. *The Man Who Mistook His Wife for a Hat and Other Clinical Tales.* New York: Harper and Row.

Sankar, Andrea. 1991. *Dying at Home: A Family Guide for Caregiving.* Baltimore: Johns Hopkins University Press.

Shaffer, Martin. 1982. *Life after Stress.* New York: Plenum Press.

Sharp, Anne. 1986. *The Nursing Home Connection: A Handbook for Visitors.* San Diego: author.

Sheridan, Carmel. 1987. *Failure-Free Activities for the Alzheimer's Patient: A Guidebook for Caregivers.* San Francisco: Cottage Books.

Ship, Jonathan A. 1992. Oral Healthy Patients with A.D. *Journal of the American Dental Association*, 123:Jan.

Shorter, Edward. 1991. Historical Changes in the Subjective Experience of Alzheimer's Disease: The Role of Anxiety. *American Journal of Alzheimer's Care and Related Disorders and Research*, 35–39:May/June.

Sloane, Philip D., and Mathew, Laura J., eds. 1991. *Dementia Units in Long-Term Care*. Baltimore: Johns Hopkins University Press.

Smedes, Lewis B. 1982. *How Can It Be All Right When Everything Is All Wrong?* New York: Pocket Books.

Smith, Kerri S. 1992. *Caring for Your Aging Parents: A Source Book of Timesaving Techniques and Tips*. Lakewood, Colo.: American Source Books.

Stehman, Jean Mason; Glenner, Joy; and Neubauer, Judi. 1991. The University of California, San Diego, Continuing Medical Education and the Alzheimer's Family Centers School of Dementia Care Training Program for Licensed Residential Care Facilities for the Elderly. *American Journal of Alzheimer's Care and Related Disorders and Research*, 6:15–18.

St. George-Hyslop, P. H. 1994. The Molecular Genetics of Alzheimer's Disease. In *Alzheimer Disease*, ed. R. D. Terry, R. Katzman, and K. L. Bick. New York: Raven Press.

Stephens, Mary Ann; Crowther, Janis H.; Hobfoll, Steven E.; and Tennenbaum, Daniel L. 1990. *Stress and Coping in Later-Life Families*. New York: Hemisphere.

Strachan, Geraldine I., and Glenner, George G. 1996. Delirium, Dementia, and Amnesic and Other Cognitive Disorders. In *Psychiatric Mental Health Nursing*, ed. K. M. Fortinash and P. A. Holoday-Warret. St. Louis: Mosby.

Taira, Ellen D. 1986. *Therapeutic Interventions for the Person with Dementia*. Binghamton, N.Y.: Haworth Press.

Tanner, Frederika. 1989. *Blueprint for a Specialized Alzheimer's Disease Nursing Home: Recommendations for Policy Planning, Patient Care, and Architectural Design*. Boston: Massachusetts Alzheimer's Disease Research Center.

Tellis-Nayak, V., and Tellis-Nayak, Mary. 1989. Quality of Care and the Burden of Two Cultures: When the World of the Nurse's Aide Enters the World of the Nursing Home. *Gerontological Society of America* 29:307–13.

Tepper, Lynn M., and Toner, John A. 1993. *Respite Care: Programs, Problems, and Solutions*. Philadelphia: Charles Press.

Terry, R. D., Katzman, R., and Bick, K. L., eds. 1994. *Alzheimer Disease*. New York: Raven Press.

Thews, Vikki; Reaves, Antonia; and Henry, Rona, eds. 1993. *Now What? A Handbook of Activities for Adult Day Programs*. Winston-Salem, N.C.: Bowman Gray School of Medicine, Wake Forest University.

Thomas, Clayton L. 1993. *Tabers Cyclopedic Medical Dictionary*, 17th ed. Philadelphia: F. A. Davis.

Tideiksaar, Rein. 1993. Preventing Bed Falls. *Nursing Update* 4:Spring.

Tornatore, Frank L. 1993. Drug Therapy. *Long-Term Care Quality Letter* 5:Feb.

U.S. Congress, Office of Technology Assessment. 1987. *Losing a Million Minds: Confronting the Tragedy of Alzheimer's Disease and Other Dementias*. Pub. no. OTA-BA-323. Washington, D.C.: Government Printing Office.

———. 1992. *Special Care Units for People with Alzheimer's and Other Dementias: Consumer Education, Research, Regulatory, and Reimbursement Issues*. Pub. no. OTA-H-543. Washington, D.C.: Government Printing Office.

U.S. Department of Health and Human Services, Public Health Service, National Institutes of Health. 1987. Differential Diagnosis of Dementing Disease. *National Institutes of Health Consensus Development Conference Statement* 6:11.

————. 1992. *Urinary Incontinence in Adults: Clinical Practice Guideline.* AHCPR Pub. no. 92-0038. Rockville, Md.: Agency for Health Care Policy and Research.

————, National Institute on Aging. 1993. *Resource Directory for Older People.* NIH Pub. no. 93-738. Bethesda, Md.: National Institute on Aging.

United States Pharmacopeial Convention. 1991. *Drug Information for the Health Care Professional,* Vols. 1A and 1B. Rockville, Md.: United States Pharmacopeial Convention.

Verdell, Lisa, and John Bouda. 1990. *Resource Guide to Continence Products and Services.* Union, S.C.: Help for Incontinent People.

Walsh, Margaret, with assistance of Berson, Ann. 1992. *Resolving the Dilemmas of the Difficult-to-Serve: Innovative Strategies and Training Techniques.* Washington, D.C.: Foundation for Hospice and Home Care.

Weissert, William G.; Elston, Jennifer M.; Bolda, Elise J.; Zelman, William N.; Mutran, Elizabeth; and Mangum, Anne B. 1990. *Adult Day Care: Findings from a National Survey.* Baltimore: Johns Hopkins University Press.

Will, Connie A., and Eighmy, Judith. 1983. *Being a Long-Term Care Nursing Assistant,* 3d ed. Englewood Cliffs, N.J.: Brady Regents / Prentice Hall.

Wolman, Benjamin B. 1973. *Dictionary of Behavioral Science.* New York: Van Nostrand Reinhold.

Zarit, Steven H. 1980. *Aging and Mental Disorders: Psychological Approaches to Assessment and Treatment.* New York: Free Press.

Zgola, Jitka M. 1987. *Doing Things: A Guide to Programing Activities for Persons with Alzheimer's Disease and Related Disorders.* Baltimore: Johns Hopkins University Press.

Zgola, Jitka. 1990. Alzheimer's Disease and the Home: Issues in Environmental Design. *American Journal of Alzheimer's Care and Related Disorders and Research,* 15–22:May / June.